AIR FRY

COOKBOOK

Series 5

This Book Includes : "Air Fryer Cookbook + The Essential Air Fryer Recipes"

By Denise White and Marisa Smith

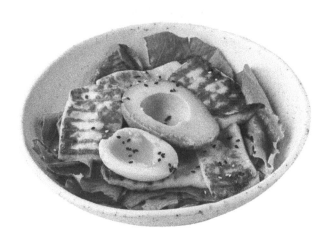

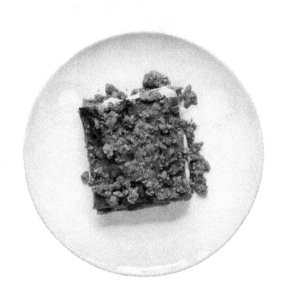

AIR FRYER COOKBOOK

Table of Contents

THE ESSENTIAL AIR FRYER RECIPES

Table of Contents

Air Fryer Cookbook

100 Quick, Easy and Delicious Affordable Recipes for beginners

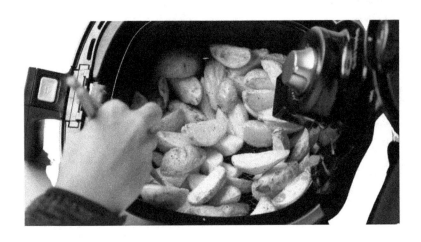

By Marisa Smith

Introduction

Air fryers use dry air and less oil to cook your food. As per an estimation, 40 calories are found per teaspoon of oil (120 calories per tablespoon). The small amount of fat you add makes the results all too delicious and extra crispy to brown and caramelize. The amount you can see in the air fryer is basically nothing compared to the amount of oil in deep-fried foods, contributing to fewer calories than the normal fried food when saturated fat. The benefits of using an air freezer actually outweigh the risks. Besides that, the food turns out crispy and crunchy.

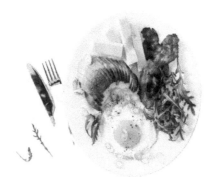

Air Fryer Recipes

1.Squash Oat Muffins

Total time: 30 min

Prep time: 10 min

Cook time: 20 min

Yield: 12 servings

Ingredients:

- Two eggs
- 1 tbsp. pumpkin pie spice
- 2 tsp. baking powder
- 1 cup oats
- 1 cup all-purpose flour
- 1 tsp. vanilla
- 1/3 cup olive oil
- 1/2 cup yogurt
- 1/2 cup maple syrup
- 1 cup butternut squash puree
- 1/2 tsp. sea salt

Directions:

1. Strip 12 cups of a cupcake muffin tin with liners.

2. Wire rack insertion at rack position 6. Pick bake, set temperature to 390 f, 20-minute timer. To preheat the oven, press start.

3. Whisk together the milk, vanilla, oil, yogurt, maple syrup, and squash puree in a large bowl.

4. Mix together the rice, pumpkin pie spice, baking powder, oatmeal and salt in a shallow dish.

5. Apply the mixture of flour to the mixture and whisk to blend.

6. Scoop the batter and bake it for 20 minutes in a prepared muffin tin.

7. Enjoy and serve.

2.Hash brown Casserole

Total time: 1 hour 10 min

Prep time: 10 minutes

Cook time: 60 minutes

Yield: 10 servings

Ingredients:

- 32 oz. frozen hash browns with onions and peppers
- 2 cups cheddar cheese, shredded
- 15 eggs, lightly beaten
- Five bacon slices, cooked and chopped
- Pepper
- Salt

Directions:

1. Spray 9*13-inch casserole dish with cooking spray and set aside.
2. Insert wire rack in rack position 6. Select bake, set temperature 350 f, timer for 60 minutes. Press start to preheat the oven.
3. In a large mixing bowl, whisk eggs with pepper and salt. Add 1 cup cheese, bacon, and hash browns and mix well.
4. Pour egg mixture into the prepared casserole dish and sprinkle with remaining cheese.
5. Bake for 60 minutes or until the top is golden brown.
6. Slice and serve.

3.Mexican Breakfast Frittata

Prep time: 10 minutes

Cook time: 25 minutes

Yield: 6 servings

Ingredients:

- 8 eggs, scrambled
- 1/2 cup cheddar cheese, grated
- 3 scallions, chopped
- 1/3 lb. tomatoes, sliced
- 1 green pepper, chopped
- 1/2 cup salsa
- 2 tsp. taco seasoning
- 1 tbsp. olive oil
- 1/2 lb. ground beef
- Pepper
- Salt

Directions:

1. Spray a baking dish with cooking spray and set it aside.
2. Insert wire rack in rack position 6. Select bake, set temperature 375 f, timer for 25 minutes. Press start to preheat the oven.
3. Heat oil in a pan over medium heat. Add ground beef to a pan and cook until brown.
4. Add salsa, taco seasoning, scallions, and green pepper into the pan and stir well.
5. Transfer meat into the prepared baking dish. Arrange tomato slices on top of the meat mixture.
6. In a bowl, whisk eggs with cheese, pepper, and salt. Pour egg mixture over meat mixture and bake for 25 minutes.
7. Serve and enjoy.

4.Perfect Brunch Baked Eggs

Total time: 30 min

Prep time: 10 minutes

Cook time: 20 minutes

Servings: 4

Ingredients:

- 4 eggs
- 1/2 cup parmesan cheese, grated
- 2 cups marinara sauce
- Pepper
- Salt

Directions:

1. Spray with cooking spray on four shallow baking dishes and set aside.

2. Wire rack insertion at rack position 6. Pick bake, set temperature to 390 f, 20-minute timer. To preheat the oven, press start.

3. Divide the marinara sauce into four plates for baking.

4. Through each baking dish, split the egg. Sprinkle the eggs with cheese, pepper, and salt and bake for 20 minutes.

5. Enjoy and serve.

5. Green Chile Cheese Egg Casserole

Prep time: 10 minutes

Cook time: 40 minutes

Yield: 12 servings

Ingredients:

- 12 eggs
- 8 oz. can green chilies, diced
- 6 tbsp. butter, melted
- 3 cups cheddar cheese, shredded
- 2 cups curd cottage cheese
- 1 tsp. baking powder
- 1/2 cup flour
- Pepper
- Salt

Directions:

1. Spray a 9*13-inch baking dish with cooking spray and set aside.

2. Insert wire rack in rack position 6. Select bake, set temperature 350 f, timer for 40 minutes. Press start to preheat the oven.

3. In a large mixing bowl, beat eggs until fluffy. Add baking powder, flour, pepper, and salt.

4. Stir in green chilies, butter, cheddar cheese, and cottage cheese.

5. Pour egg mixture into the prepared baking dish and bake for 40 minutes.

6. Slice and serve.

6.Kale Zucchini Bake

Prep time: 10 minutes

Cook time: 30 minutes

Yield: 4 servings

Ingredients:

- 1 onion, chopped
- 1 cup zucchini, shredded and squeezed out all liquid
- 1/2 tsp. dill
- 1/2 tsp. oregano
- Six eggs
- 1 cup cheddar cheese, shredded
- 1 cup kale, chopped
- 1/2 tsp. basil
- 1/2 tsp. baking powder
- 1/2 cup almond flour
- 1/2 cup milk
- 1/4 tsp. salt

Directions:

1. With cooking oil, spray a 9*9-inch baking dish and put it aside.

2. Wire rack insertion at rack position 6. Pick bake, set temperature to 375 f, 35-minute timer. To preheat the oven, press start.

3. Whisk the eggs with the milk in a large mixing cup. Add the remaining ingredients, stirring until well mixed.

4. In the prepared baking dish, add in the egg mixture and bake for 35 minutes.

5. Slicing and cooking.

7.Cheesy Breakfast Casserole

Total time: 1 hour 10 min

Prep time: 10 min

Cook time: 60 min

Yield: 6 servings

Ingredients:

- 4 eggs
- 2 cups of milk
- 1 1/2 cup cheddar cheese, shredded
- Five bread slices, cut into cubes
- Pepper
- Salt

Directions:

1. Spray one 1/2-quart of baking dish and set aside with cooking spray.

2. Layer cubes of bread and alternately shredded cheese in a prepared baking dish.

3. Whisk the eggs with sugar, pepper and salt in a bowl and spill over the bread mixture. Put in the refrigerator overnight with a baking bowl.

4. Insert wire rack in place of rack 6. Pick bake, set temperature to 350 f, 60-minute timer. To preheat the oven, press start.

5. Take the baking dish out of the oven. For 60 minutes, roast.

6. Slicing and cooking.

8.Easy Hash Brown Breakfast Bake

Total time: 55 min

Prep time: 10 min

Cook time: 45 min

Yield: 8 servings

Ingredients:

- 8 eggs
- 1 cup cheddar cheese, shredded
- 1 lb. bacon slices, cooked and crumbled
- Pepper
- 30 oz. frozen cubed hash brown potatoes, thawed
- 2 cups of milk
- Salt

Directions:

1. Spray a 13*9-inch baking dish with cooking spray and set aside.
2. Insert wire rack in rack position 6. Select bake, set temperature 350 f, timer for 45 minutes. Press start to preheat the oven.
3. Add hash brown, bacon, and 1/2 cup cheese into the prepared baking dish.
4. In a bowl, whisk eggs with milk, pepper, and salt and pour over hash brown mixture. Sprinkle with remaining cheese and bake for 45 minutes.
5. Slice and serve.

9.Mexican Chiles Breakfast Bake

Total time: 50 min

Prep time: 10 min

Cook time: 40 min

Yield: 15 servings

Ingredients:

- Six eggs
- 20 oz. hash brown potatoes, shredded
- 1/4 tsp. ground cumin
- 1/2 cup milk
- 2 cups Mexican cheese, shredded
- 1 lb. pork sausage, cooked and crumbled
- 1 cup chunky salsa
- 28 oz. can whole green chilies
- Pepper
- Salt

Directions:

1. Spray a 13*9-inch baking dish with cooking spray and set aside.
2. Insert wire rack in rack position 6. Select bake, set temperature 350 f, timer for 40 minutes. Press start to preheat the oven.
3. Layer half potatoes, chilies, salsa, half sausage, and half cheese into the prepared baking dish. Cover with remaining sausage, potatoes, and cheese.
4. In a bowl, whisk eggs with milk, cumin, pepper, and salt and pour over potato mixture and bake for 40 minutes.
5. Serve and enjoy.

10.Delicious Amish Baked Oatmeal

Total time: 40 min

Prep time: 10 min

Cook time: 30 min

Yield: 8 servings

Ingredients:

- Two eggs
- 3 cups rolled oats

- 1 tsp. cinnamon
- 1 1/2 tsp. vanilla
- 1 1/2 tsp. baking powder
- 1/4 cup butter, melted
- 1/2 cup maple syrup
- 1 1/2 cups milk
- 1/4 tsp. salt

Directions:

1. Spray an 8*8-inch baking dish with cooking spray and set aside.
2. Insert wire rack in rack position 6. Select bake, set temperature 350 f, timer for 30 minutes. Press start to preheat the oven.
3. In a large bowl, whisk eggs with milk, cinnamon, vanilla, baking powder, butter, maple syrup, and salt. Add oats and mix well.
4. Pour mixture into the baking dish and bake for 30 minutes.
5. Slice and serve with warm milk and fruits.

11.Pork Sirloin Steak

Total time: 55 min

Prep time: 40 min

Cook time: 15 min

Yield: 2 servings

Ingredients:

- 1/2 onion
- 1 teaspoon ginger powder
- 1 teaspoon garlic powder
- 1 teaspoon ground cinnamon
- 1/2 teaspoon ground cardamom
- 1/2 - 1 teaspoon cayenne
- 1 teaspoon salt

- 1-pound boneless pork sirloin steaks

Directions:

1. Start by seasoning the steaks with pork loin. A generous amount of black pepper and salt, with a slight sprinkle of dried sage, is all you want to use. Don't be shy when it comes to seasoning. Before proceeding, making sure to season all sides of all the steaks properly.

2. On medium to high heat, melt a tablespoon of butter in a skillet. I want to wait until the cooking and bubbling of the butter begins. This means that the entire pan is heavy. This recipe for pork loin steak requires butter, not cooking spray or grease. Cooking steaks in butter adds so much flavor to them, and I notice that juicy steaks are created in this way.

3. It's time to add the steaks when the pan is heated, and the butter is melting and fried. You can cook 1 or 2 of them at a time. Just make sure you're not overfilling your plate. Leave it to cook until faint signs of browning begin to surface on the underside, then turn and cook on the other side. This is 4-5 minutes of cooking time on either side.

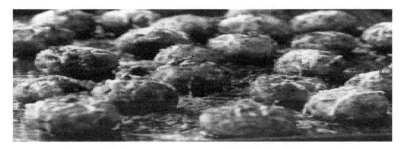

12.Chicken Meatballs with Cream Sauce and Cauliflower

Prep time: 40 min

Cook time: 15 min

Yield: 2 servings

Ingredients:

- 10 oz. Ground chicken
- 1 egg
- 2 oz. Grated parmesan cheese
- 1 teaspoon salt
- ½ teaspoon pepper
- 1 teaspoon dried basil
- 2 tablespoons sun-dried tomatoes in oil
- 1 tablespoon butter
- 1 lb. cauliflower
- 2 tablespoons butter for serving
- Cream sauce
- 1¼ cups coconut cream
- 1 tablespoon tomato paste
- 3 tablespoons finely chopped
- Fresh basil

Directions:

1. Combine the ground chicken ingredients and use a spoon to make 10 to 12 large balls (per pound). Following the manufacturer's instructions, ready the fryer. With a paper towel, gently coat the basket with elongated coconut oil and bake at 350 degrees for 10-13 minutes until lightly browned. Bring the oven back in and cook for another 4 to 5 minutes.

2. Place it on a plate after frying, then apply the cream and tomato paste. Let it cook over medium heat for 10 minutes.

3. With salt and pepper, season. Just before serving, add the fresh basil and cook the cauliflower for a few minutes in gently salted water. Serve alongside the chicken balls and cream sauce with a spoonful of sugar.

13.Shrimp Salad

Total time: 25 min

Prep time: 10 min

Cook time: 15 min

Yield: 2 servings

Ingredients:

- The salad
- 6 leaves lettuce
- 300 grams peeled shrimp
- 1 ½ tablespoon avocado oil
- ½ cup chopped celery
- 1 stalk chopped leek
- 4 tablespoons Greek yogurt
- 1 tablespoon coconut cream
- ½ teaspoon mint
- ½ teaspoon dried basil
- ¼ teaspoon chili powder
- 1 teaspoon lime juice

Directions:

1. Place the shrimp in the frying basket in one layer and air fried in the oven at 400 ° f for 10-14 minutes, depending on the size of the shrimp.

2. In a cup, mix together Greek yogurt, coconut milk, mint, dried basil, chili powder and lime juice.

3. Using the sliced celery and leek to place the fried shrimp in the dish. Combine the shrimp and vegetables before the dressing is covered.

4. Divide the lettuce and fill with the salad into separate portions.

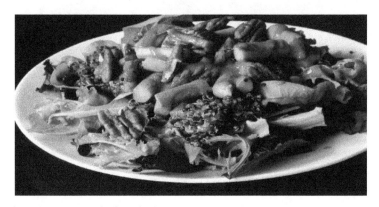

14.Maple Asparagus Salad with Pecans

Total time: 25 min

Prep time: 10 min

Cook time: 15 min

Yield: 4 servings

Ingredients:

- 10 medium asparagus spears
- ½ cup cherry tomatoes halved
- ½ cup chopped pecans
- ½ cup crumbled feta cheese
- 1-1/2 tablespoons coconut oil
- 1 tablespoon maple syrup

Directions:

1. Clean and cut the rough ends of the asparagus and spray coconut oil on the asparagus.

2. In an air fryer, place the asparagus in the oven. Cook at 360 degrees for 6 to 10 minutes to be crispy. In a cup, put the tomato halves, the diced pecans and the grated feta cheese.

3. In a shallow bowl, combine the coconut oil with the maple syrup and add the asparagus to the salad mix. Pour over the salad with the dressing combination.

4. To ensure the ingredients are evenly covered, combine the lettuce.

15.Creamed Kale

Total time: 25 min

Prep time: 10 min

Cook time: 15 min

Yield: 4 servings

Ingredients:

- 1 10 ounces package frozen kale, thawed
- 1/2 cup onions, chopped
- 2 teaspoons garlic powder
- 4 ounces cream cheese, diced
- 1 teaspoon ground black pepper
- 1 teaspoon salt
- 1/2 teaspoon ground cinnamon
- 1/4 cup shredded goat cheese

Directions:

1. Grease a 6-inch pan and set it aside. Mix the kale, onion, garlic, diced cream cheese, salt, pepper and cinnamon in a medium bowl.

2. Pour into a greased pan and place the fryer at 350 ° f for 10 minutes. Open and mix the kale to mix the goat cheese through the kale and sprinkle the goat over it.

3. Set the fryer to 400 ° f for 5 minutes or until the cheese melts and turns brown.

16.Baked Zucchini

Total time: 25 min

Prep time: 10 min

Cook time: 15 min

Yield: 4 servings

Ingredients:

- 2 medium-large zucchinis

- 1 teaspoon coconut oil
- 2 teaspoons butter
- 1 teaspoon stevia
- 1/2 teaspoon nutmeg

Directions:

4. Rub the zucchinis with olive oil

5. Place the zucchinis in the air fryer. Cook for 40 minutes at 400 degrees.

6. Remove the zucchinis from the air fryer and allow them to cool.

7. Slice them open and load 1 teaspoon of butter and stevia and 1/4 teaspoon of nutmeg into each.

8. Cooking time may vary because every air fryer brand is different.

17.Roasted Broccoli Avocado Soup

Total time: 20 min

Prep time: 10 min

Cook time: 10 min

Yield: 4 servings

Ingredients:

- 1 head broccoli
- 1 tablespoon garlic powder
- 2 cups chicken stock or vegetable stock
- 1 avocado peeled and cubed
- 1/2 lemon juiced
- 1 tablespoon coconut oil
- Sea salt to taste
- Fresh ground pepper to taste

Directions:

9. Preheat the fryer to 390 degrees. Mix broccoli with garlic powder, salt and pepper and roast for 10 minutes. Carefully pour the broccoli with

the other ingredients into the blender at high speed and puree until it is smooth.

10. Add salt and pepper as desired, add water too thin to desired consistency if necessary and heat slightly over medium heat. Serve immediately.

18. Herbed Tuna

Total time: 20 min

Prep time: 10 min

Cook time: 10 min

Yield: 2 servings

Ingredients:

- 8 oz. Sizzle fish tuna filets
- 1 teaspoon herbs
- 1/4 teaspoon sea salt
- 1/4 teaspoon black pepper
- 1/4 teaspoon smoked paprika
- 2 tablespoons coconut oil
- 1 tablespoon butter

Directions:

1. Using a paper towel to dry fillets and run the surface carefully to ensure there are no bones.

2. Spray the fish with coconut oil and brush it on the two sides of the solution.

3. On both sides of the fish, combine the seasoning and scatter.

4. Cook an air fryer for 5-8 minutes at 390 degrees. Starting with 5 minutes, I suggest testing the fish and adding another minute to the time before it quickly crumbles with a fork.

5. In the oven, heat the seasoned butter for 30 seconds and spill it over the fish before eating.

19. Sirloin Steak

Total time: 20 min

Prep time: 10 min

Cook time: 10 min

Yield: 2 servings

Ingredients:

- 2 sirloin steaks
- Two tablespoons steak seasoning
- Coconut oil

Directions:

1. Using a paper towel to dry fillets and run the surface carefully to ensure there are no bones.

2. Spray the fish with coconut oil and brush it on the two sides of the solution.

3. On both sides of the fish, combine the seasoning and scatter.

4. Cook an air fryer for 5-8 minutes at 390 degrees. Starting with 5 minutes, I suggest testing the fish and adding another minute to the time before it quickly crumbles with a fork.

5. In the oven, heat the seasoned butter for 30 seconds and spill it over the fish before eating.

20. Whole Chicken

Total time: 1 hour 5 min

Prep time: 05 min

Cook time: 60 min

Yield: 4 servings

Ingredients:

- 1 (4-pound) whole chicken,
- 1 tablespoon coconut oil
- ¼ tablespoon kosher salt
- ½ teaspoon freshly ground black pepper
- ½ teaspoon garlic powder
- ½ teaspoon paprika (I prefer smoked paprika)
- ¼ teaspoon dried mint
- ¼ teaspoon dried oregano

- ¼ teaspoon dried thyme

Directions:

1. Mix all of the spices into a paste with the oil and spread them all over the chicken.

2. Spray a basket of air fryers with an oil spray. Place the chicken in the basket face down and cook for 50 minutes at 360f.

3. Turn the chicken upside down and cook 10 minutes more.

4. Verify that there is an internal temperature of 165f in the breast chicken. Slice and serve.

21. Mini Sweet Pepper Poppers

Total time: 30 min

Prep time: 10 min

Cook time: 20 min

Yield: 4 (2 per servings)

Ingredients:

- 8 mini sweet peppers
- 4 ounces of full-Fat: cream cheese, softened
- 4 slices of sugar-free bacon, cooked and crumbled
- 1/4 cup of shredded pepper jack cheese

Directions:

1. Cut the pepper tops and slice on half lengthwise each. To cut seeds and membranes using a small knife.

2. Put together the cream cheese, bacon, and pepper jack in a shallow bowl.

3. In each sweet pepper, put 3 teaspoons of the mixture and press smoothly hard—place in basket fryer.

4. Set the temperature to 400° F, and set the timer for eight minutes.

5. Serve and enjoy!

22. Spicy Spinach Artichoke Dip

Total time: 30 min

Prep time: 10 min

Cook time: 20 min

Yield: (2 per servings)

Ingredients:

- 10 ounces of frozen spinach, drained and thawed
- 1 (14-ounce) can of artichoke hearts, drained and chopped
- 1/4 cup of chopped pickled jalapenos
- 8 ounces of full-Fat: cream cheese, softened
- 1/4 cup of full-Fat: mayonnaise
- 1/4 cup of full-Fat: sour cream
- 1/2 teaspoon of garlic powder
- ¼ cup of grated Parmesan cheese
- 1 cup of shredded pepper jack cheese

Directions:

1. In a 4-cup baking dish, combine the ingredients. In the Air Fryer, bring the basket in.
2. Fix the temperature for 10 minutes to 320° F and adjust the timer.
3. Start with an orange, then a bubble. Serve new and savor it!

23.Personal Mozzarella Pizza Crust

Total time: 30 min

Prep time: 10 min

Cook time: 20 min

Yield: (1per servings)

Ingredients:

- 1/2 cup of shredded whole-milk mozzarella cheese
- 2 tablespoons of blanched finely ground almond flour
- 1 tablespoon of full-Fat: cream cheese
- 1 large egg white

Directions:

1. In a medium microwave-safe bowl, place the mozzarella, almond flour, and cream cheese. Microwave that lasted 30 seconds. Stir until the dough ball forms smoothly. Add egg white and stir until the dough forms soft and round.

2. Press the crust of a 6 round pizza.

3. Cut a piece of parchment to fit your Air Fryer basket and place the crust on the parchment.

4. Set the temperature to 350° F and adjust the timer for 10 minutes.

5. Flip over the crust after 5 minutes and place any desired toppings at this time. Continue to cook until golden. Serve immediately.

24.Garlic Cheese Bread

Total time: 20 min

Prep time: 10 min

Cook time: 10 min

Yield: (2per servings)

Ingredients:

- 1 cup of shredded mozzarella cheese
- 1/4 cup of grated Parmesan cheese
- 1 large egg
- 1/2 teaspoon of garlic powder

Directions:

1. In a wide bowl, combine the ingredients. To suit your Air Fryer basket, cut a piece of parchment. Press the mixture in a circle onto the parchment, and put it in the Air Fryer basket.

2. Fix the temperature for 10 minutes to 350° F and adjust the timer.

3. Serve it warm and eat it!

25.Crustless Three-Meat Pizza

Total time: 20 min

Prep time: 10 min

Cook time: 10 min

Yield: (2per servings)

Ingredients:

- 1/2 cup of shredded mozzarella cheese
- 7 slices of pepperoni
- 1/4 cup of cooked ground sausage
- 2 slices of sugar-free bacon, cooked and crumbled
- 1 tablespoon of grated Parmesan cheese
- 2 tablespoons of low-carb, sugar-free pizza sauce for dipping

Directions:

1. Cover the bottom of the cake pan with mozzarella. Put the pepperoni, sausage, and bacon on top of the cheese and sprinkle with the Parmesan. Place the pan in the basket of the Air Fryer.

2. Change the temperature to 400° F and set a 5-minute timer.

3. Cut until the cheese is crispy and bubbling. Serve warm with a pizza sauce for dipping.

26.Smoky BBQ Roasted Almonds

Total time: 20 min

Prep time: 10 min

Cook time: 10 min

Yield: (2per servings)

Ingredients:

- 1 cup of raw almonds
- 2 teaspoons of coconut oil
- 1 teaspoon of chili powder
- 1/4 teaspoon of cumin
- 1/4 teaspoon of smoked paprika
- 1/4 teaspoon of onion powder

Directions:

1. Put all the ingredients in a big bowl before the almonds are filled equally with oil and spices. Put the almonds in the Air Fryer box.

2. Fix the temperature for 6 minutes to 320° F and adjust the timer.

3. Halfway through the cooking process, remove the basket from the fryer. Enable it to totally cool off.

27.Beef Jerky

Total time: 20 min

Prep time: 10 min

Cook time: 10 min

Yield: (2per servings)

Ingredients:

- 1-pound of flat iron beef, thinly sliced
- 1/4 cup of soy sauce
- 2 teaspoons of Worcestershire sauce
- 1/4 teaspoon of crushed red pepper flakes
- 1/4 teaspoon of garlic powder
- 1/4 teaspoon of onion powder

Directions:

1. Place all the ingredients in a plastic bag or sealed container and marinate for 2 hours in the fridge.

2. On the Air Fryer rack, placed each jerky slice into a single sheet.

3. Fix the temperature to 160° F and for 4 hours, set the timer.

4. Up to 1 week of storage in airtight containers.

28.Pork Rind Nachos

Total time: 20 min

Prep time: 10 min

Cook time: 10 min

Yield: (2per servings)

Ingredients:

- 1-ounce of pork rinds

- 4 ounces of shredded cooked chicken
- 1/2 cup of shredded Monterey jack cheese
- 1/4 cup of sliced pickled jalapeños
- 1/4 cup of guacamole
- 1/4 cup of full-Fat: sour cream

Directions:

In a 6' round baking tray, put pork rinds. Fill with grilled chicken and cheese jack from Monterey. Place the Air Fryer in the basket with the plate.

Set the temperature to 370 degrees F and set the timer before the cheese is melted or for 5 minutes.

With jalapeños, guacamole, and sour cream, enjoy right now.

29.Ranch Roasted Almonds

Total time: 20 min

Prep time: 10 min

Cook time: 10 min

Yield: (2per servings)

Ingredients:

- 2 cups of raw almonds
- 2 tablespoons of unsalted butter, melted
- 1/2 (1-ounce) ranch dressing mix packet

Directions:

1. To coat equally, stir the almonds in a large bowl of butter. Place almonds in the basket for Air Fryer Sprinkle ranch blend and sprinkle over almonds.
2. Fix the temperature for 6 minutes to 320° F and adjust the timer.
3. Shake the basket two or three times during training.
4. For at least 20 minutes, let it cool down. Almonds can become smooth during refrigeration to become crunchier. Place it in an air-tightened container for up to 3 days.

30.Loaded Roasted Broccoli

Total time: 20 min

Prep time: 10 min

Cook time: 10 min

Yield: (2per servings)

Ingredients:

- 3 cups of fresh broccoli florets
- 1 tablespoon of coconut oil
- 1/2 cup of shredded sharp Cheddar cheese
- 1/4 cup of full-Fat: sour cream
- 4slices of sugar-free bacon, cooked and crumbled
- 1 scallion, sliced

Directions:

1. Take the broccoli and drizzle it with coconut oil in the Air Fryer bowl.
2. Switch the temperature to 350 degrees F and set the timer for a further 10 minutes.
3. During exercise, toss a basket two or three times, or stop burning spots.
4. Remove from the fryer as the top begins to crisp the broccoli. Garnish with the melted cheese, sour cream, and crumbled bacon and scallion slices.

31.Scrumptious Leg of Lamb

Preparation time: 5 minutes

Cooking time: 1 hour

Servings: 4

Ingredients:

- 1 1/4 kg leg of lamb
- 1 tablespoon olive oil

- A pinch of sea salt
- Pepper

Directions:

1. Season the lamb's leg with salt and pepper and put it in the basket of the fryer.

2. Cook at 360 degrees for 20 minutes, turn the lamb's leg over and cook for a further 20 minutes.

3. Using roasted potatoes to serve.

32.Chinese Style Pork Chops

Preparation time: 15 minutes

Cooking time: 20 minutes

Servings: 4

Ingredients:

- 450g Pork chops
- ¾ cup corn/potato starch
- 1 egg white
- ¼ tsp. Freshly ground black pepper
- ½ tsp. Kosher salt
- For the stir fry:
- 2 green onions, sliced
- 2 jalapeno peppers, seeds removed and sliced
- 2 tbsp. Peanut oil
- ¼ tsp. Freshly ground pepper and kosher salt to taste

Directions:

1. Brush or spray with oil on the basket of your toast oven air fryer.

2. Next, mix the egg, salt and black pepper until it's frothy. Break up the pork chops and wipe the meat dry using a clean kitchen towel.

3. Toss the cutlets until evenly covered in the frothy egg mixture. For 30 minutes, cover and marinate.

4. Place the pork chops in a separate bowl and pour in the starch of corn/potato to ensure that each culet is dredged thoroughly. Shake off the extra corn/potato starch and place the prepared basket with the pork chops.

5. Set the air fryer toast oven to 360 degrees F and cook for 9 minutes, then shake the basket every 2-3 minutes, and if necessary, spray or brush the cutlets with more oil.

6. Increase the temperature to 400 degrees F and cook for another 6 minutes or until the chops are crisp.

7. Heat a wok or pan until incredibly hot over high heat. Apply all the ingredients for the stir fry and sauté for a minute.

8. Attach the pork chops you've fried and toss them with the stir fry.

9. Cook for another minute to guarantee that the stir-fry ingredients are uniformly mixed with the pork chops.

Enjoy!

33.Cinco De Mayo Pork Taquitos

Preparation time: 20 minutes

Cooking time: 15 minutes

Servings: 5

Ingredients:

- 400g cooked and shredded pork tenderloin
- 10 flour tortillas2 ½ cups mozzarella, shredded
- 1 lemon, juiced
- Sour cream
- Salsa
- Cooking spray

Directions:

1. Set your air fryer toast oven to 380 degrees f.

2. Squeeze the lemon juice over the shredded pork and mix well to combine.

3. Divide the tortillas into two and microwave, I batch at a time, covered with a slightly damp paper towel, so they don't become hard, for 15 seconds.

4. Divide the pork and cheese among the 10 tortillas.

5. Gently but tightly roll up all the tortillas.

6. Line your air fryer toast oven's pan with kitchen foil and arrange the tortillas on the pan.

7. Spray the tortillas with the cooking spray and cook for about 10 minutes, turning them over halfway through cook time.

8. Serve hot and enjoy!

34.Tangy Smoked Pork Chops with Raspberry Sauce

Preparation time: 15 minutes

Cooking time: 25 minutes

Servings: 4

Ingredients:

- 4 medium-sized smoked pork chops
- 1 cup panko bread crumbs
- 2 eggs
- ¼ cup all-purpose flour
- ¼ cup milk
- 1 cup pecans, finely chopped
- 1/3 cup aged balsamic vinegar
- 2 tbsp. Raspberry jam, seedless
- 1 tbsp. Orange juice concentrate
- 2 tbsp. Brown sugar

Directions:

1. Set your air fryer toast oven to 400 degrees f and spray/brush your air fryer toast oven's basket gently with oil.

2. Combine the milk and the eggs using a fork.

3. Mix the panko bread crumbs with the finely diced pecan in a separate bowl and place the flour in a third bowl.

4. Coat, one chop of pork at a time, of starch, brushing off the surplus.

5. Next, dunk the milk mixture and gently coat the crumb mixture on both sides. Gently pat to make the crumbs bind to the pork chops.

6. In the prepared basket, place the pork chops in one layer, spray lightly with cooking oil and cook for about 15 minutes, turning the chops halfway through the cooking time.

7. Combine all of the remaining ingredients in a pan over low-medium heat while the chops are frying. Carry to a boil until it thickens, then cook for 5-8 minutes.

8. Take out the chops and serve hot with the raspberry sauce.

9. Enjoy!

35.Air fryer toast oven bacon

Preparation time: 5 minutes

Cooking time: 15 minutes

Servings: 6

Ingredients:

- 1/2 package (16 ounces) bacon

Directions:

1. Preheat to 390° f with your air fryer toast cooker.

2. Arrange the bacon in the basket of the fryer in a single layer and cook for 8 minutes.

3. Flip the bacon over and cook for 7 more minutes or until crisp.

4. To drain excess grease, move it to a paper-lined tray.

5. Enjoy warm!

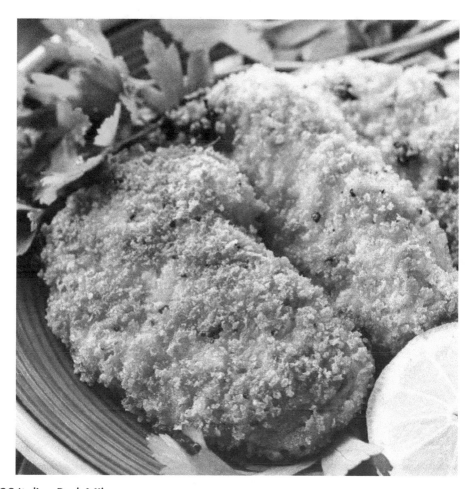

36.Italian Pork Milanese

Preparation time: 20 minutes

Cooking time: 10 minutes

Servings: 46

Ingredients:

- 6 pork chops, center-cut
- 2 eggs
- 2 tbsp. Water
- 1 cup panko bread crumbs seasoned with salt and black pepper
- ½ cup all-purpose flour

- 2 tbsp. Extra virgin olive oil

- Parmesan cheese, for serving (optional)

- For arugula salad:

- 1 bag fresh arugula

- 2 tbsp. Freshly squeezed lemon juice

- 1 tsp. Dijon mustard

- 1/8 cup extra virgin olive oil

- Freshly ground black pepper and sea salt to taste

Directions:

1. To pound each chop of pork into 1/4 inch cutlets, use a mallet or rolling pin.

2. Season well with salt and pepper, then dip the flour into each cutlet. Shake the waste off.

3. In a small cup, whisk the eggs with water and dip the floured cutlets in the mixture, then roll them into the bread crumbs.

4. For all of the chops, do this and put it aside.

5. Set 380 degrees f for your air fryer toast oven.

6. Brush the breaded pork chops gently with olive and place the toast oven basket in one sheet on your air fryer. Cook for 3-5 minutes or until golden and crisp, then flip the chops and cook for another 3-5 minutes.

7. Meanwhile, in a large bowl, cook the salad by mixing the mustard, lemon juice, salt and pepper. With the vinaigrette, toss the arugula until finely covered.

8. Serve the arugula salad and top with crisp cutlets and parmesan cheese (optional). Enjoy!

37.Jamaican Jerk Pork Roast

Preparation time: 10 minutes

Cooking time: 1 hour 10 minutes

Servings: 10

Ingredients:

- 1800g pork shoulder
- 1 tbsp. Olive oil
- 1/4 cup Jamaican jerk spice blend
- 1/2 cup beef broth

Directions:

1. Set your air fryer to 400 degrees f and brown roast on both sides for 4 minutes on each side after rubbing the oil and seasoning.

2. Then decrease the temperature to 350 degrees f and bake for 1 hour, then remove from the fryer.

3.

4. Shred and serve.

38.Tasty and Moist Air Fryer Toast Oven Meatloaf

Preparation time: 20 minutes

Cooking time: 20 minutes

Servings: 4

Ingredients:

- 450 g lean minced meat
- 250 ml tomato sauce
- 1 small onion, finely chopped
- 1 tsp. Minced garlic
- 5 tbsp. Ketchup
- 1 tbsp. Worcestershire sauce
- 1/3 cup cornflakes crumbs
- 3 tsp. Brown sugar
- 1 ½ tsp. Freshly ground black pepper

- 1 ½ tsp. Sea salt
- 1 tsp. Dried basil
- ½ tsp. Freshly chopped parsley

Directions:

1. Combine the minced beef, corn flakes, chopped onion, garlic, basil, salt, pepper, and 3/4 of the tomato sauce in a large bowl. To blend and ensure that all the ingredients are mixed equally, use your hands.

2. Take your two shallow loaf pans and brush them loosely with vegetable oil. Divide the mixture of the meatloaf into two loaf pans.

3. Set the oven to 360 degrees f for your air fryer breakfast.

4. Combine the remainder of the tomato sauce, ketchup, Worcestershire sauce and brown sugar in a cup for the glaze. On the top and sides of the two loaves, rub this glaze blend.

5. Place the loaf pans, too, in the fryer. Cook and re-apply the glaze on the top and sides of the meatloaves for 10 minutes.

6. Cook for a further 10 minutes, twice in between, adding the glaze.

7. Sprinkle with the new parsley and cut the two loaf pans.

8. Before extracting the loaves from the loaf pans, let them stand for 3 minutes.

9. With mashed potatoes and a green salad, serve the perfectly moist and delicious meatloaf.

10. Enjoy!

39.Classic Country Fried Steak

Preparation time: 15 minutes

Cooking time: 20 minutes

Servings: 2

Ingredients:

- 2 x 200g sirloin steaks
- 1 cup panko bread crumbs seasoned with kosher salt and freshly ground pepper
- 1 cup all-purpose flour
- 3 eggs, lightly beaten
- 1 tsp. Garlic powder
- 1 tsp. Onion powder
- For the sausage gravy:
- 150g ground sausage meat
- 2 cups milk
- 2 ½ tbsp. Flour
- 1 tsp. Freshly ground black pepper

Directions:

11. To pound the two steaks up to 1/2 - 1/4 inches thick, use a mallet or rolling pin.

12. In three separate shallow containers, placed the flour, egg and panko.

13. Dredge the steak in the flour first, then the egg and finally the bread crumbs then set them aside on a pan.

14. Brush the basket gently with oil from your air fryer toast oven, and then put the two breaded steaks on the basket.

15. Set the oven to 370 degrees f for the air fryer toast and cook the steak for 12 minutes, flipping once halfway through the cooking time.

16. Meanwhile, prepare the gravy by frying the sausage meat over medium-low heat in a pan until it browns uniformly. Drain the extra fat and reserve it in the pan for around a tablespoon or two.

17. Stir in the flour until well mixed, then, little by little, pour in the milk, stirring all the while.

18. For 3 minutes, season with freshly ground pepper and boil until the gravy is good and thick.

19. Using the sauce and some fluffy mashed potatoes to eat the steak. Yum!

40. Bourbon Infused Bacon Burger

Preparation time: 45 minutes

Cooking time: 30 minutes

Servings: 2

Ingredients:

- 300g 80:20 lean ground beef
- 3 strips maple bacon, halved
- 1 small onion, minced
- 1 tbsp. Bourbon
- 2 tbsp. Bbq sauce
- 2 tbsp. Brown sugar
- 2 slices Monterey jack cheese
- Freshly ground black pepper, to taste
- Salt, to taste
- 2 burger rolls
- Sliced tomato for serving
- Torn lettuce, for serving
- For the sauce:
- 2 tbsp. Mayonnaise
- 2 tbsp. Bbq sauce
- ¼ tsp. Sweet paprika

- Freshly ground black pepper, to taste

Directions:

1. Set your air fryer toast oven to 390 degrees F and pour around 1/2 cup of water into your air fryer toast oven's bottom drawer. This causes the smoking/burning grease to trickle away.

2. Mix the bourbon with the sugar. Arrange the strips of bacon in the basket of your air fryer toast oven and spray the tops with the sugar-bourbon mixture. Cook for 4 minutes, change the strips and brush with more sugar-bourbon mix and cook until brown and super crisp for 4 more minutes.

3. Meanwhile, the ground beef, chopped onion, salt, pepper and bbq sauce are mixed to create the burgers. To mix well, use your hands to make 2 burger patties.

4. If you like your burgers well cooked, set the air fryer toast oven at 370 degrees f and cook the burgers for 20 minutes, or 12-15 minutes if you like them medium-rare. Halfway into cooking time, flip the burgers.

5. Meanwhile, mix all the sauce ingredients in a bowl and stick them in the fridge to produce the sauce.

6. Cover each burger with a slice of Monterey Jack cheese for one minute of your cooking time. To keep the cheese from being blown away in the fryer, bind the cheese to the patty using a toothpick.

7. Cut each roll and spread the sauce on the sliced halves of the rolls to assemble the burger. Place one half of the burger and cover it with the bacon, tomatoes, lettuce and the other half of the roll. Enjoy!

41.Glazed Lamb Chops

Preparation time: 10 minutes

Cooking time: 15 minutes

Servings: 4

Ingredients:

- 1 tablespoon dijon mustard
- ½ tablespoon fresh lime juice
- 1 teaspoon honey
- ½ teaspoon olive oil
- Salt and ground black pepper, as required
- 4 (4-ounce) lamb loin chops

Directions:

1. In a black pepper large bowl, mix the mustard, lemon juice, oil, honey, salt, and black pepper.
2. Add the chops and coat with the mixture generously.
3. Place the chops onto the greased "sheet pan."
4. Press the "power button" of the ninja food digital air fry oven and turn the dial to select the "air bake" mode.
5. Press the time button and again turn the dial to set the cooking time to 15 minutes.
6. Now push the temp button and rotate the dial to set the temperature at 390 degrees f.
7. Press the "start/pause" button to start.
8. When the unit beeps to show that it is preheated, open the lid.
9. Insert the "sheet pan" in the oven.
10. Flip the chops once halfway through.
11. Serve hot.

42.Buttered Leg of Lamb

Preparation time: 15 minutes

Cooking time: 1¼ hours

Servings: 8

Ingredients:

- 1 (2¼-pound) boneless leg of lamb
- 3 tablespoons butter, melted
- Salt and ground black pepper, as required
- 4 fresh rosemary sprigs

Directions:

1. Rub with butter on the leg of the lamb and sprinkle with salt and black pepper.
2. Wrap a leg of lamb with sprigs of rosemary.
3. "Press the ninja foodie digital air fry oven's "power button" and turn the dial to select the mode for "air fry.
4. To set the cooking time to 75 minutes, press the time button and change the dial once again.
5. Now press the temp button to set the temperature at 300 degrees f and rotate the dial.
6. To start, press the 'start/pause' button.
7. "Open the "air fry basket" lid and grease when the machine beeps to indicate that it is preheated.
8. Arrange the leg of lamb into an "air fry basket" and insert it in the oven.
9. Remove from the oven and put the lamb's leg on a cutting board before slicing for about 10 minutes.
10. Split into bits of the appropriate size and serve.

43.Glazed Lamb Meatballs

Preparation time: 20 minutes

Cooking time: 30 minutes

Servings: 8

Ingredients:

- For meatballs:
- ½ cup Ritz crackers, crushed
- Salt and ground black pepper, as required
- 1 (5-ounce) can evaporate milk
- 2 large eggs, beaten lightly
- 1 tablespoon dried onion, minced
- 1 teaspoon maple syrup
- 2 pounds lean ground lamb
- 2/3 cup quick-cooking oats
- For sauce:
- 1/3 cup sugar
- 1/3 cup orange marmalade
- 1-2 tablespoons sriracha
- 1/3 cup maple syrup
- 1 tablespoon Worcestershire sauce
- 2 tablespoons cornstarch
- 2 tablespoons soy sauce

Directions:

1. For meatballs: Put all the ingredients in a large bowl and mix until well mixed.
2. From the mixture, produce 11/2-inch balls.
3. Add half of the meatballs in a single layer to the greased "sheet pan."
4. "Press the ninja foodie digital air fry oven's "power button" and turn the dial to select the mode for "air fry.
5. To set the cooking time to 15 minutes, click the time button and change the dial once again.
6. Now press the temp button to set the temperature at 380 degrees f and rotate the dial.

7. To start, press the 'start/pause' button.

8. Open the lid when the device beeps to demonstrate that it is preheated.

9. Place the' sheet pan' in the oven.

10. Halfway through, turn the meatballs once.

11. Remove the meatballs from the oven and transfer them to a dish.

12. Repeat with the meatballs that remain.

13. Meanwhile, for sauce, put all the ingredients in a small pan: over medium heat and cook until thickened, stirring constantly.

14. Serve the meatballs with sauce on top.

44.Oregano Lamb Chops

Preparation time: 10 minutes

Cooking time: 30 minutes

Servings: 4

Ingredients:

- 4 lamb chops
- 1 garlic clove, peeled
- 1 tbsp. plus
- 2 tsp. olive oil
- ½ tbsp. oregano
- ½ tbsp. thyme
- Salt and black pepper to taste

Directions:

1. Preheat the fryer to 390 f for air. Coat the clove of garlic with 1 tsp. Place the olive oil in the air fryer for 10 minutes. Meanwhile, with the remaining olive oil, combine the herbs and seasonings.

2. Squeeze the hot roasted garlic clove into the herb mixture using a towel or a mitten, and stir to blend. Cover the lamb chops well with the mixture and put them in the oven for frying. For 8 to 12 minutes, cook. Serve it warm.

45.Lamb Steaks with Fresh Mint and Potatoes

Preparation time: 10 minutes

Cooking time: 25 minutes

Servings: 2

Ingredients:

- 2 lamb steaks
- 2 tbsp. Olive oil
- 2 garlic cloves, crushed
- Salt and pepper, to taste
- A handful of fresh thyme, chopped
- 4 red potatoes, cubed

Directions:

1. Using oil, garlic, salt, and black pepper to rub the steaks. In the fryer, put the thyme and place the steaks on top. Oil the chunks of the potato and sprinkle them with salt and pepper. Arrange the potatoes next to the steaks and cook for 14 minutes at 360 f, turning once halfway through the cooking process.

46.Lamb Kofta

Preparation time: 6 minutes

Cooking time: 12 minutes

Servings: 4

Ingredients:

- 1 pound ground lamb
- 1 tsp. cumin
- 2 tbsp. mint, chopped
- 1 tsp. garlic powder
- 1 tsp. onion powder
- 1 tbsp. ras el hanout
- ½ tsp. ground coriander

- 4 bamboo skewers
- Salt and black pepper to taste

Directions:

2. Lamb, cumin, garlic powder, mint, onion powder, ras el hanout, cilantro, salt and pepper are combined in a cup. Place on skewers and mold into sausage shapes. Marinate it in the fridge for 15 minutes.

3. Preheat to 380 f with your air fryer. Spray a basket of air fryers with cooking spray. Arrange the skewers in the basket of an air fryer. Cook for 8 minutes, turning once halfway through. Serve with dip with yogurt.

47.Crunchy Cashew Lamb Rack

Preparation time: 10 minutes

Cooking time: 30 minutes

Servings: 4

Ingredients:

- 3 oz. chopped cashews
- 1 tbsp. chopped rosemary
- 1 ½ lb. rack of lamb
- 1 garlic clove, minced
- 1 tbsp. breadcrumbs
- 1 egg, beaten
- 1 tbsp. olive oil
- Salt and pepper to taste

Directions:

1. Heat the air-freezer to 210 f. Combine the garlic with the olive oil and spray this mixture over the lamb. In a dish, blend the rosemary, cashews, and crumbs. Brush the lambs with the egg, then cover them with the cashew mixture. Place the lamb in the basket of an air fryer and cook for 25 minutes. Increase the heat to 390 f, and cook for an additional 5 minutes. Cover with foil and leave to rest before serving for a few minutes.

48.Oregano & Thyme Lamb Chops

Preparation time: 10 minutes

Cooking time: 30 minutes

Servings: 4

Ingredients:

- 4 lamb chops
- 1 garlic clove, peeled
- 1 tbsp. plus
- 2 tsp. olive oil
- ½ tbsp. oregano
- ½ tbsp. thyme
- ½ tsp. salt
- ¼ tsp. black pepper

Directions:

2. Preheat the fryer to 390 f for air. Coat the clove of garlic with 1 tsp. Olive oil and put for 10 minutes in the air fryer. With the remaining olive oil, combine the herbs and seasonings.

3. Squeeze the hot roasted garlic clove into the herb mixture using a towel or a mitten, and stir to blend. Thoroughly coat the lamb chops with the mixture, and put in the air fryer. 12 minutes to cook.

49.Lamb Meatballs

Preparation time: 10 minutes

Cooking time: 40 minutes

Servings: 12

Ingredients:

- 1 ½ lb ground lamb
- ½ cup minced onion
- 2 tbsp. chopped mint leaves
- 3 garlic cloves, minced

- 2 tsp. paprika
- 2 tsp. coriander seeds
- ½ tsp. cayenne pepper
- 1 tsp. salt
- 1 tbsp. chopped parsley
- 2 tsp. cumin
- ½ tsp. ground ginger

Directions:

20. Soak 24 skewers in water until ready to use. Preheat the air fryer to 330 f. Combine all ingredients in a large bowl. Mix well with your hands until the herbs and spices are evenly distributed, and the mixture is well combined. Shape the lamb mixture into 12 sausage shapes around 2 skewers. Cook for 12 to 15 minutes, or until it reaches the preferred doneness. Served with tzatziki sauce and enjoy.

50.Thyme Lamb Chops with Asparagus

Preparation time: 10 minutes

Cooking time: 20 minutes

Servings: 4

Ingredients:

- 1 pound lamb chops
- 2tspolive oil
- 1½ tsp. chopped fresh thyme
- 1 garlic clove, minced
- Salt and black pepper to taste
- 4 asparagus spears, trimmed

Directions:

1. Preheat to 400 f with your air fryer. Spray a basket of air fryers with cooking spray.

2. Drizzle some olive oil with the asparagus, sprinkle with salt, and set aside with salt and black pepper, season the lamb. Brush and move

the remaining olive oil to the cooking basket. Slide the basket out, transform the chops and add the asparagus. Cook for 10 minutes. For another 5 minutes, cook. Serve with thyme sprinkles.

51.Cornflakes French toast

Total time: 20 min

Prep time: 10 min

Cook time: 10 min

Yield: 2 servings

Ingredients:

- Bread slices (brown or white)
- 1 egg white for every 2 slices
- 1 tsp. of sugar for every 2 slices
- Crushed cornflakes

Directions:

1. Place two slices together, then trim them along the diagonal. In a bowl, whisk together the egg whites, then add a little sugar.
2. Immerse the bread triangles in this mixture and coat them with the crushed corn blossoms.
3. Preheat the Air Fryer at 180o C for 4 minutes. Place the triangles of coated bread in and close the box for frying. Let them cook for at least a further 20 minutes at the same temperature.
4. To get an even chef, turn the triangles over. Serve the slices of chocolate syrup.

52.Mint Galette

Total time: 10 min

Prep time: 5 min

Cook time: 5 min

Yield: 2 servings

Ingredients:

- 2 cups of mint leaves (Sliced fine)

- 2 medium potatoes boiled and mashed
- 1 ½ cup of coarsely crushed peanuts
- 3 tsp. of ginger finely chopped
- 1-2 tbsp. of fresh coriander leaves
- 2 or 3 green chilies finely chopped
- 1 ½ tbsp. of lemon juice
- Salt and pepper to the taste

Directions:

1. Mix the sliced mint leaves with the remaining ingredients in a clean dish. Shape this mixture into galettes that are flat and round.

2. Wet the galettes softly with sweat. Cover each peanut with each smashed galette.

3. Preheat the Air Fryer, at 160° Fahrenheit, for 5 minutes. Place the galettes in the frying bowl and let them steam at about the same temperature for another 25 minutes.

4. In order to get a cook that is even, keep turning them over. Using chutney, basil, or ketchup to serve.

53.Cottage Cheese Sticks

Total time: 10 min

Prep time: 5 min

Cook time: 5 min

Yield: 2 servings

Ingredients:

- 2 cups of cottage cheese
- 1 big lemon-juiced
- 1 tbsp. of ginger-garlic paste

For seasoning, use salt and red chili powder in small amounts

- ½ tsp. of carom
- One or two papadums

- 4 or 5 tbsp. of cornflour
- 1 cup of water

Directions:

1. Take the cheese and cut it into pieces that are long. Currently, a combination of lemon juice, red chili powder, spices, ginger garlic paste, and caramel is used as a marinade.

2. Marinate the slices of cottage cheese in the mixture for a bit, then wrap them in dry cornflour for about 20 minutes to set aside.

3. Take the papadum and cook it in a saucepan. Crush them until they are cooked into very tiny pieces. Take another bottle now and pour about 100 ml of water in it.

4. Loosen 2 tablespoons of cornflour in the water. Dip the cottage cheese pieces in this cornflour solution and roll them on to the bits of crushed papadum so that the papadum attaches to the cottage cheese.

5. Preheat the Air Fryer for 10 minutes at about 290 Fahrenheit. Then open the basket for the fryer and put the cottage cheese bits inside it. Cover the bowl well. Enable the fryer to sit at 160 ° for another 20 minutes.

6. Open the basket halfway through, and put a little of the cottage cheese around to allow for standard cooking. Until they're cooked, you can eat them with either ketchup or mint chutney. Serve and chutney with mint.

54.Palak Galette

Total time: 20 min

Prep time: 10 min

Cook time: 10 min

Yield: 2 servings

Ingredients:

- 2 tbsp. of garam masala
- 2 cups of Palak leaves
- 1 ½ cup of coarsely crushed peanuts

- 3 tsp. of ginger finely chopped
- 1-2 tbsp. of fresh coriander leaves
- 2 or 3 green chilies finely chopped
- 1 ½ tbsp. of lemon juice
- Salt and pepper to the taste

Directions:

1. Blend into a clean container with the ingredients. Shape this mixture into galettes that are smooth and round. Wet the galettes softly with sweat. Coat up each galette with smashed peanuts.

2. Preheat the Air Fryer, at 160° Fahrenheit, for 5 minutes. Place the galettes in the basket and let them cook for another 25 minutes at the same temperature. Go turn them over to cook them. Using ketchup or mint chutney to serve.

55.Spinach Pie

Total time: 10 min

Prep time: 5 min

Cook time: 5 min

Yield: 2 servings

Ingredients:

- 7 ounces of flour
- 2 tablespoons of butter
- 7ounces of spinach
- 1 tablespoon of olive oil
- 2 eggs
- 2 tablespoons of milk
- 3 ounces of cottage cheese
- Salt and black pepper to the taste
- 1 yellow onion, chopped

Directions:

1. In your food processor, mix flour and butter, 1 egg, milk, salt and pepper, combine properly, switch to a cup, knead, cover, and leave for 10 minutes.

2. Heat the pan with the oil over medium heat, add the spinach and onion, stir and simmer for 2 minutes.

3. Attach salt, pepper, cottage cheese, and leftover egg, stir well and heat up.

4. Divide the dough into 4 pieces, roll each piece, place it on a ramekin's rim, add the spinach filling over the dough, place the ramekins in your Air Fryer's basket, and cook at 360° F for 15 minutes.

5. Serve it sweet.

56. Balsamic Artichokes

Total time: 10 min

Prep time: 5 min

Cook time: 5 min

Yield: 7 servings

Ingredients:

- 4 big artichokes, trimmed
- Salt and black pepper to the taste
- 2 tablespoons of lemon juice
- ¼ cup of extra virgin olive oil
- 2 teaspoons of balsamic vinegar
- 1 teaspoon of oregano, dried
- 2 garlic cloves, minced

Directions:

1. Season the salt and pepper with the artichokes, rub them with half the oil and half the lemon juice, put them in your Air Fryer and cook at 360 ° F for 7 minutes.

2. Meanwhile, in a cup, combine the remaining lemon juice, vinegar, remaining oil, salt, pepper, garlic, and oregano and mix well.

3. Arrange the artichokes on a tray, coat them with a balsamic vinaigrette, and eat.

57.Cheesy Artichokes

Total time: 15 min

Prep time: 5 min

Cook time: 5 min

Yield: 7 servings

Ingredients:

- 14 ounces of canned artichoke hearts
- 8 ounces of cream cheese
- 16 ounces of parmesan cheese, grated
- 10 ounces of spinach
- ½ cup of chicken stock
- 8 ounces of mozzarella, shredded
- ½ cup of sour cream
- 3 garlic cloves, minced
- ½ cup of mayonnaise
- 1 teaspoon of onion powder

Directions:

1. In a saucepan appropriate for your Air Fryer, blend artichokes with stock, garlic, spinach, cream cheese, sour cream, onion powder and mayo, put in the Air Fryer, and cook for 6 minutes at 350 °F.
2. Apply the mozzarella and parmesan and then stir well and eat.

58.Artichokes and Special Sauce

Total time: 15 min

Prep time: 5 min

Cook time: 5 min

Yield: 2 servings

Ingredients:

- 2 artichokes, trimmed
- A drizzle of olive oil
- 2 garlic cloves, minced
- 1 tablespoon of lemon juice

For the sauce:

- ¼ cup of coconut oil
- ¼ cup of extra virgin olive oil
- 3 anchovy fillets
- 3 garlic cloves

Directions:

1. Mix the artichokes with the oil, 2 cloves of garlic and lemon juice in a cup, toss well, move to your Air Fryer, and cook for 6 minutes at 350 ° F and split between plates.
2. Mix coconut oil with anchovy, 3 garlic cloves, and olive oil in your food processor, blend very well, drizzle with artichokes and eat.

59.Beet Salad and Parsley Dressing

Total time: 25 min

Prep time: 10 min

Cook time: 25 min

Yield: 4 servings

Ingredients:

- 4 beets
- 2 tablespoons of balsamic vinegar
- A bunch of parsley, chopped
- Salt and black pepper to the taste
- 1 tablespoon of extra-virgin olive oil
- 1 garlic clove, chopped
- 2 tablespoons of capers

Directions:

1. Place the beets and cook at 360 ° F for 14 minutes in your Air Fryer.

2. Meanwhile, in a dish, mix the parsley, garlic, salt, pepper, olive oil, and capers, and whisk very well.

3. Move the beets to a cutting board, cool them down, slice them, and place them in a salad bowl.

4. All over the parsley dressing, apply vinegar and drizzle and eat.

60.Beets and Blue Cheese Salad

Total time: 25 min

Prep time: 10 min

Cook time: 25 min

Yield: 6 servings

Ingredients:

- 6 beets, peeled and quartered

- Salt and black pepper to the taste

- ¼ cup of blue cheese, crumbled

- 1 tablespoon of olive oil

Directions:

1. In the Air Fryer, place the beets, cook them at 350 ° F for 14 minutes and then move them to a dish.

2. Apply the blue cheese, salt, pepper, and oil to the mixture, and then toss and eat.

61.Shrimp Pancakes

Preparation Time: 5 Minutes

Cooking Time: 15 Minutes

Servings: 10-12

Ingredients:

- 1 cup all-purpose flour

- 1 glass of water

- 3 beaten eggs

- 1 tablet chicken broth

Directions:

1. Boil the water and dissolve the chicken broth, let it cool and place the beaten eggs and the wheat flour, stir well until everything dissolves and a smooth mass fry the tablespoons and a little oil in the Tefal pan and keep the part in a baking dish.

2. Make the prawns taste and leave with a little sauce.

3. Top with pancakes and shrimp sauce and sprinkle with grated cheese. Do this until the last layers of grated cheese are ready.

4. Bake in the air fryer at 3600F for 15 minutes. Serve with white rice and salad.

62.Shrimps with Palmito

Preparation Time: 10 Minutes

Cooking Time: 30 Minutes

Servings: 4-8

Ingredients:

White Sauce:

- 1 cup grated Parmesan cheese
- 1 tbsp. butter
- 4 ½ lb shrimp
- ½ cup of olive oil
- Very minced garlic Striped onion
- 1 can of sour cream
- 1 can of sliced palm heart Grated Parmesan

Sauce:

- 1 onion, sliced
- Margarine and butter
- 2 cups milk
- 2 tbsp. of flour
- Salt to taste

- cheese for sprinkling

Preparation of the white sauce:

1. With the margarine and butter, lightly brown the onion.

2. In a blender, place the milk and wheat flour.

3. Add the onion which has been stewed.

4. Beat it all really well.

5. Bring this mixture to the fire and cook until a dense cream appears. Add the Parmesan cheese and butter and extract the white sauce from the heat. Reserve. Reserve.

6. Sauté the snails with garlic and onion in olive oil.

7. To the white sauce, add the sautéed shrimp and eventually add the palm kernel and milk, mixing it all very well.

8. Sprinkle plenty of Parmesan cheese on top, set in a greased refractory form.
9. Bake for 1520 minutes in the air-fryer at 3600F.

63.Gratinated Pawns with Cheese
Preparation Time: 10 Minutes

Cooking Time: 20 Minutes

Servings: 4

Ingredients:

- 2 ¼ lbs. clean, chopped prawns
- 1 tbsp. of fondor
- 1 tbsp. of oil
- 1 tbsp. butter
- 1 grated onion
- 5 tomatoes, beaten in a blender
- 1 tablet of crumbled shrimp broth
- 1 glass of light cream cheese
- 1 tbsp. of breadcrumbs
- 1 tbsp. Parmesan cheese

Directions:

1. Use one such fondor to season the prawns and reserve for 1 hour.

2. In the oil and butter combination, cook them.

3. Position them and set them aside in a refractory container.

4. Brown, the onion in the fat of the shrimp, add the tomatoes, a tablet of the shrimp broth and a cup of boiling water.

5. Bring to a boil, until just a touch, in a covered skillet.

6. Add the curd, then stir until it freezes.

7. Pour over the prawns and sprinkle the mixed breadcrumbs with the grated rib.

8. Parmesan cheese and placed it in a 400oF air fryer for 20 minutes or until golden brown.

64.Air fryer Crab
Preparation Time: 5 Minutes

Cooking Time: 10 Minutes

Servings: 20

Ingredients:

- 1 pound of crab meat 20 crab cones
- 2 onions
- 2 tomatoes
- 3 garlic cloves
- 1 bell pepper
- ½ glass of white vinegar
- 1 head of black pepper
- 1 head of cumin
- 1 small salt
- Olive oil to taste

Directions:

1. Place the onion that has been sliced until golden. Then, with 1/2 glass of vinegar, add the remaining spices (pepper, cumin, minced garlic).

2. Put in the green smell, the crushed tomatoes, and the cut pepper. Add the olive oil to taste when the seasoning is well done (at least 3 tablespoons).

3. Then add the meat to the crab and cook for 5 minutes.

4. Fill the crab cones, drizzle with grated Parmesan cheese and bake for 5 minutes in an air fryer at 3200 to melt the cheese.

65.Crab Balls

Preparation Time: 10 Minutes

Cooking Time: 20 Minutes

Servings: 2-4

Ingredients:

- 1 lb of crab Salt to taste Olive oil
- 2 cloves garlic, minced
- 1 chopped onion
- 3 tbsp. of wheat flour
- 1 tbsp. of parsley
- 1 fish seasoning
- 2 lemons
- 1 cup milk

Tarnish:

1. Wash the crab in the juice of 1 lemon.

2. Season with the juice of the other lemon, along with the salt and the prepared fish seasoning.

3. In a frying pan, sauté the onion and garlic with the sweet oil.

4. Mix the crab meat with the stir fry. 5. Let cook in this mixture for another 5 minutes.

6. Add the parsley.

7. Dissolve the flour in the milk and add it to the crab.

8. Stir constantly, until this mixture begins to come out of the pan.

9. Let cool, shape the meatballs, go through the beaten egg and breadcrumbs.

10. 1 beaten egg Bread crumbs Oil for frying

11. Fry in the air fryer at 4000F for 25 minutes.

66.Crab Empanada

Preparation Time: 15 Minutes

Cooking Time: 30 Minutes

Servings: 4-8

Ingredients:

- 1 small onion
- 1 tomato
- 1 small green pepper
- 1 lb of crab meat Seasoning ready for fish
- 1 tbsp. of oil Pastry dough

Directions:

1. In oil, sauté the chopped onion, tomato, and pepper.

2. Add the sauce and crab meat.

3. Cook, without stirring, until very dry so that it does not stick to the bottom of the pan.

4. Fill the cakes with the crab meat that has been prepared.

5. Fry it in an air fryer for 25 minutes at 4000F.

67.Crab Meat on Cabbage

Preparation Time: 10 Minutes

Cooking Time: 15 Minutes

Servings: 2-4

Ingredients:

- 1 pound shredded crab meat
- 1 pound cooked and minced dogfish

- 2 cups of cooked rice
- 1 small green cabbage
- Parsley and coriander
- Chile
- 2 tbsp. of palm oil

Directions:

1. In a little water, season and cook the dogfish.

2. Crush the broth that has been created when it is smooth and drink it. Add the crab meat, which should have been thawed already. Add the tomato sauce, palm oil, pepper and cooked rice.

3. In warm water, dissolve the starch and pour it into the mixture. Sharpen the mixture, taste the salt and brush on top with the chopped parsley and coriander.

4. Cook 6 whole leaves of cabbage separately, until al dente, in salted water.

5. Place the open leaves and crab cream with 2 tbsp. of cornstarch in a baking dish. Tomato sauce Bread crumbs Garlic fish inside.

7. Sprinkle with breadcrumbs and bake for 5 minutes in an air fryer at 3200F to brown.

68.Gratinated Cod

Preparation Time: 15 Minutes

Cooking Time: 45 Minutes

Servings: 4-8

Ingredients:

- 2 ¼ lb cod
- 1 red bell pepper
- 1 green bell pepper
- 1 onion
- 3 ripe tomatoes
- 2 cloves of garlic
- 1 cup black olives

- Oregano to taste

Cream:

- 1 cup catupiry cheese
- 1 can of cream
- ½ cup coconut milk

Mashed potatoes:

1. First, prepare the mashed potatoes, squeeze the potatoes and, with the potatoes still very sweet, add the butter and cream, mix well and add salt to taste.

2. On a high ovenproof plate, put this puree. Then arrange yourself like a pie crust. Make the stir fry with the already desalted cod (soak the day before and change the water at least 5 times).

3. Bring to a boil briefly, in boiling water, for 5 minutes.

4. Crush the cod into chips, then.

5. In a frying pan, put ample oil and cook the onion and garlic. Then add 2 1/4 lb of boiled and squeezed potatoes 2 butter spoons 1/2 cup of milk Salt to taste Sour cream and bell peppers and simmer for about 10 minutes.

6. Then add the cod and olives and let it simmer for 10 further minutes.

7. Without letting so much of it dry out. And, to taste, apply oregano. You don't usually have to add salt since the cod already contains plenty of it.

8. If you need to bring in a bit, however.

9. Play over mashed potatoes with this braised cod. Cream:: Cream

10. In a blender, beat all the ingredients and pour over the cod.

11. For 30 minutes or until it is orange, take it to the previously heated air fryer at 6000F.

12. Serve with a leafy salad and white rice.

69.Gratinated Cod with Vegetables
Preparation Time: 10 Minutes

Cooking Time: 30 Minutes

Servings: 2-4

Ingredients:

- 2 ¼ lb cod 1 pound of potato 1 pound carrot
- 2 large onions
- 2 red tomatoes
- 1 bell pepper
- 1 tbsp. of tomato paste
- Coconut milk
- Garlic, salt, coriander and olive oil to taste.
- Olives

Sauce:

1. For 24 hours, soak the cod, always changing the water. Blanch, removing skin and pimples, at a fast boil. Strain and reserve the water where the cod has been cooked.

2. Season the French fries with cod, garlic, salt and coriander. On top of that, put a saucepan with olive oil and sliced onions on the fire. Add the onions, pepper, and chopped olives, skinless and seedless. Mix in the cod, tomato extract, coconut milk, and a little water to prepare the cod. Let them all cook a lot. There was a lot of sauce moving on. Get the salt tested. Sliced potatoes and carrots are cooked.

3. In a blender, whisk together milk, wheat and 2 cups milk 1 1/2 tablespoons all-purpose flour 1 tablespoon butter 1 egg 1/2 cup sour cream Nutmeg, black pepper and melted salt butter. Bring it to the fire and stir until it thickens the mixture. Finally, add the milk, nutmeg, black pepper, beaten egg and salt.

4. After rubbing a clove of garlic inside, grease a plate with olive oil. In alternate layers, arrange the cod, potato, and carrot. Cover all with sauce and bake for 20 minutes in an air fryer at 3800F.

70.Salmon Fillet

Preparation Time: 10 Minutes

Cooking Time: 15 Minutes

Servings: 2-4

Ingredients:

- 1 lb salmon fillet

- Sliced pitted olives
- Oregano
- 3 tbsp. soy sauce
- Salt to taste
- Olive oil to taste
- Lemon
- Aluminum foil
- ½ sliced onion

Directions:

1. Wash the salmon with lemon juice.

2. Heat the oil and add the sliced onion, leaving it on the fire until it becomes transparent. Reservation.

3. Cover a baking sheet with aluminum foil so that leftovers can cover all the fish.

4. In the foil on the baking sheet, place the fish already seasoned with salt, drizzle with olive oil and soy sauce.

5. Garnish with sliced olives and a little oregano. Pour the onion on top. Wrap with aluminum foil so that the liquid does not spill when it starts to heat up.

6. Bake in the air fryer at 4000F for about 30 minutes.

7. Serve with vegetables and green salad.

71.Hake Fillet with Potatoes
Preparation Time: 10 Minutes

Cooking Time: 30 Minutes

Servings: 2-4

Ingredients:

- 8 fillets of hake
- 4 raw potatoes
- 1 bell pepper
- 2 tomatoes

- 1 onion Good quality tomato sauce.
- Oregano
- Oil for greasing

Directions:

1. As desired, season the fillets and reserve for 10 minutes. Use olive oil to grease an ovenproof dish to create a coat of potato, then put the fillets on the potato. Drizzle with tomato sauce (1/2 can) and add onion, tomato, bell pepper, oregano to taste.

2. With the rest of the potatoes, seal. Cover and bake with foil until the potatoes are tender. Using lemon juice, wash the salmon. Heat the oil until it becomes transparent, and add the sliced onion, leaving it on the flames. On reservation.

3. Cover a baking sheet of aluminum foil so that all the fish can be covered with leftovers.

4. Place the fish, which is already seasoned with salt in the foil on the baking sheet, drizzle with olive oil and soy sauce.

5. Add chopped olives and a little oregano to the garnish. On top, pour the onion. Wrap the aluminum foil so that as it begins to heat up, the liquid does not leak.

6. Bake in an air-fryer for about 30 minutes at 4000F. 7. Serve with green salad and vegetables.

72.Delicious Raspberry Cobbler

Total time: 20 min

Prep time: 10 min

Cook time: 10 min

Yield: 6 serving

Ingredients:

- 1 egg, lightly beaten
- 1 cup raspberries, sliced
- 2 tsp. swerve

- 1/2 tsp. vanilla
- 1 tbsp. butter, melted
- 1 cup almond flour

Directions:

1. Place the Cuisinart oven in place 1. With the rack.
2. To the baking dish, add the raspberries.
3. Sprinkle with raspberries and sweetener.
4. In a dish, combine the almond flour, vanilla, and butter together.
5. Apply the egg to the mixture of almond flour and whisk well to blend.
6. Spread a mixture of almond flour over the sliced raspberries.
7. Set for 15 minutes to bake at 350 f. Place the baking dish in the preheated oven after five minutes.
8. Enjoy and serve.

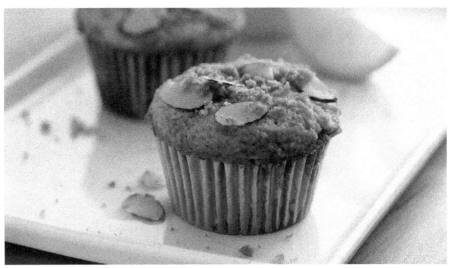

73.Orange Almond Muffins

Total time: 30 min

Prep time: 10 min

Cook time: 25 min

Yield: 2 servings

Ingredients:

- 4 eggs
- 1 tsp. baking soda
- 1 orange zest
- 1 orange juice
- 1/2 cup butter, melted
- 3 cups almond flour

Directions:

1. Place the Cuisinart oven in place 1. with the rack.
2. Line and set aside 12-cups of a muffin tin with cupcake liners.
3. In a big bowl, add all the ingredients and blend until well mixed.
4. In the prepared muffin pan, pour the mixture into it.
5. Set for 25 minutes to bake at 350 f. Place the muffin tin in the preheated oven for 5 minutes.
6. Enjoy and serve.

74.Easy Almond Butter Pumpkin Spice Cookies

Total time: 30 min

Prep time: 10 min

Cook time:25 min

Yield: 6 servings

Ingredients:

- 1/4 tsp. pumpkin pie spice
- 1 tsp. liquid Stevie
- 6 oz. almond butter
- 1/3 cup pumpkin puree

Directions:

1. Place the Cuisinart oven in place 1. with the rack.

2. In the food processor, add all ingredients and process until simply combined.

3. Into the parchment-lined baking tray, drop spoonsful of mixture.

4. Set to bake for 23 minutes at 350 f. Place the baking pan in the preheated oven after five minutes.

5. Enjoy and serve.

75. Moist Pound Cake

Total time: 40 min

Prep time: 15 min

Cook time: 25 min

Yield: 2 serving

Ingredients:

- 4 eggs
- 1 cup almond flour
- 1/2 cup sour cream
- 1 tsp. vanilla
- 1 cup monk fruit sweetener
- 1/4 cup cream cheese
- 1/4 cup butter
- 1 tsp. baking powder
- 1 tbsp. coconut flour

Directions:

1. Place the Cuisinart oven in place 1. With the rack.

2. Mix the almond flour, baking powder, and coconut flour together in a big bowl.

3. Add the cream cheese and butter to a separate bowl and microwave for 30 seconds. Stir well, then microwave for 30 more seconds.

4. Stir in the sour cream, sweetener, and vanilla. Only stir well.

5. Pour the mixture of cream cheese into the almond flour mixture and whisk until mixed.

6. Add the eggs one by one to the batter and stir until well mixed.

7. Pour the batter into a cake pan of prepared oil.

8. Set to bake for 60 minutes at 350 f. Place the cake pans in the preheated oven after five minutes.

9. Slicing and serving.

76.Banana Butter Brownie

Total time: 25 min

Prep time: 10 min

Cook time: 15 min

Yield: 6 serving

Ingredients:

- 1 scoop protein powder
- 2 tbsp. cocoa powder
- 1 cup bananas, overripe
- 1/2 cup almond butter, melted

Directions:

1. Place the Cuisinart oven in place 1. with the rack.

2. In the blender, add all the ingredients and blend until smooth.

3. Fill the greased cake pan with batter.

4. Set for 21 minutes to bake at 325 f. Place the cake pans in the preheated oven after five minutes.

5. Enjoy and serve.

77.Peanut Butter Muffins

Total time: 10 min

Prep time: 15 min

Cook time: 15 min

Yield: 12 serving

Ingredients:

- 1 cup peanut butter
- 1/2 cup maple syrup
- 1/2 cup of cocoa powder
- 1 cup applesauce
- 1 tsp. baking soda
- 1 tsp. vanilla

Directions:

1. Place the Cuisinart oven in place 1. with the rack.
2. Line and set aside 12-cups of a muffin tin with cupcake liners.
3. In the blender, add all the ingredients and blend until smooth.
4. Pour the blended mixture into the muffin tin you have packed.
5. Set for 25 minutes to bake at 350 f. Place the muffin tin in the preheated oven for 5 minutes.
6. Enjoy and serve.

78.Baked Apple Slices

Total time: 40 min

Prep time: 15 min

Cook time: 25 min

Yield: 6 serving

Ingredients:

- 2 apples, peel, core, and slice
- 1 tsp. cinnamon
- 2 tbsp. butter
- 1/4 cup of sugar
- 1/4 cup brown sugar
- 1/4 tsp. salt

Directions:

1. Place the Cuisinart oven in place 1. with the rack.

2. In the zip-lock container, add cinnamon, sugar, brown sugar, and salt and combine well.

3. Fill the bag with apple slices and shake until well coated.

4. Apply the apple slices to the greased 9-inch baking dish.

5. Set to bake for 35 minutes at 350 f. Place the baking dish in the preheated oven after five minutes.

6. Enjoy and serve.

79.Vanilla Peanut Butter Cake

Total time: 40 min

Prep time: 15 min

Cook time: 25 min

Yield: 8 serving

Ingredients:

- 1 1/2 cups all-purpose flour
- 1/3 cup vegetable oil
- 1 tsp. baking soda
- 1/2 cup peanut butter powder
- 1 tsp. vanilla
- 1 tbsp. apple cider vinegar
- 1 cup of water
- 1 cup of sugar
- 1/2 tsp. salt

Directions:

1. Place the Cuisinart oven in place 1. with the rack.

2. Mix the flour, baking soda, peanut butter powder, sugar and salt together in a large mixing bowl.

3. Whisk the oil, vanilla, vinegar, and water together in a small cup.

4. Pour the mixture of oil into the mixture of flour and whisk until well mixed.

5. Fill the greased cake pan with batter.

6. Set to bake for 35 minutes at 350 f. Place the cake pans in the preheated oven after five minutes

7. Cut and serve.

80.Moist Chocolate Brownies

Total time: 25 min

Prep time: 10 min

Cook time: 15 min

Yield: 6 serving

Ingredients:

- 1 1/3 cups all-purpose flour
- 1/2 tsp. baking powder
- 1/3 cup cocoa powder
- 1 cup of sugar
- 1/2 tsp. vanilla
- 1/2 cup vegetable oil
- 1/2 cup water
- 1/2 tsp. salt

Directions:

1. Place the cuisine-style oven with the rack in place 1.

2. Mix the flour, baking powder, cocoa powder, sugar and salt together in a large mixing bowl.

3. Whisk the oil, water and vanilla together in a small cup.

4. Pour the mixture of oil into the flour and blend until well mixed.

5. Pour in the greased baking dish with the batter.

6. Set to bake for 25 minutes at 350 f. Place the baking sheet in the preheated oven after five minutes.

7. Cut and serve.

81.Yummy Scalloped Pineapple

Total time: 40 min

Prep time: 10 min

Cook time: 25 min

Yield: 6 serving

Ingredients:

- 3 eggs, lightly beaten
- 8 oz. can crush pineapple, un-drained
- 2 cups of sugar
- 4 cups of bread cubes
- 1/4 cup milk
- 1/2 cup butter, melted

Directions:

1. Place the Cuisinart oven in place 1. with the rack.
2. Mix the eggs with the milk, butter, crushed pineapple, and sugar in a mixing cup.
3. To coat, add bread cubes and stir well.
4. Move the mixture to a greased dish for baking.
5. Set to bake for 40 minutes at 350 f. Place the baking dish in the preheated oven after five minutes.
6. Enjoy and serve.

82.Vanilla Lemon Cupcakes

Total time: 25 min

Prep time: 10 min

Cook time: 15 min

Yield: 6 serving

Ingredients:

- 1 egg
- 1/2 cup milk
- 2 tbsp. canola oil
- 1/4 tsp. baking soda
- 3/4 tsp. baking powder
- 1 tsp. lemon zest, grated
- 1/2 cup sugar
- 1 cup flour
- 1/2 tsp. vanilla
- 1/2 tsp. salt

Directions:

1. Place the Cuisinart oven in place 1. with the rack.
2. Line and set aside 12-cups of a muffin tin with cupcake liners.
3. Whisk the egg, vanilla, milk, oil, and sugar together in a bowl until smooth.
4. Apply the remaining ingredients and combine until mixed.
5. Load the batter into the muffin tin that has been packed.
6. Set for 20 minutes to bake at 350 f. Place the muffin tin in the preheated oven for 5 minutes.
7. Enjoy and serve.

83.Walnut Carrot Cake

Total time: 25 min

Prep time: 10 min

Cook time: 15 min

Yield: 4 serving

Ingredients:

- 1 egg
- 1/2 cup sugar

- 1/4 cup canola oil
- 1/4 cup walnuts, chopped
- 1/2 tsp. baking powder
- 1/2 cup flour
- 1/4 cup grated carrot
- 1/2 tsp. vanilla
- 1/2 tsp. cinnamon

Directions:

1. Place the Cuisinart oven in place 1. with the rack.
2. Beat the sugar and oil in a medium bowl for 1 minute. Apply the vanilla, egg and cinnamon and beat for 30 seconds.
3. Apply the remaining ingredients and stir well until mixed.
4. Pour the batter into the baking bowl, which is greased.
5. Set for 30 minutes to bake at 350 f. Place the baking dish in the preheated oven after five minutes.
6. Enjoy and serve.

84.Baked Peaches

Total time: 40 min

Prep time: 10 min

Cook time: 25 min

Yield: 6 serving

Ingredients:

- 4 freestone peaches, cut in half and remove stones
- 2 tbsp. sugar
- 8 tsp. brown sugar
- 1 tsp. cinnamon
- 4 tbsp. butter, cut into pieces

Directions:

1. Place the Cuisinart oven in place 1. with the rack.

2. In a baking dish, put the peach halves and fill each half with 1 tsp. of brown sugar.

3. Place butter on top of the halves of each peach.

4. Mix the cinnamon and sugar together and drizzle over the peaches.

5. Set for 30 minutes to bake at 375 f. Place the baking dish in the preheated oven after five minutes.

6. Enjoy and serve.

85.Cinnamon Apple Crisp

Total time: 35 min

Prep time: 10 min

Cook time: 20 min

Yield: 4 serving

Ingredients:

- 1/8 tsp. ground clove
- 1/8 tsp. ground nutmeg
- 2 tbsp. honey
- 4 1/2 cups apples, diced
- 1 tsp. ground cinnamon
- 1 tbsp. cornstarch
- 1 tsp. vanilla
- 1/2 lemon juice
- For topping:
- 1 cup rolled oats
- 1/3 cup coconut oil, melted
- 1 tsp. cinnamon
- 1/3 cup honey
- 1/2 cup almond flour

Directions:

1. Place the Cuisinart oven in place 1. with the rack.
2. Mix the apples, vanilla, lemon juice, and honey in a medium-sized dish. Sprinkle it on top of herbs and cornstarch and stir well.
3. Load the combination of apples into the greased baking bowl.
4. Mix together the coconut oil, cinnamon, almond flour, oats and honey in a small bowl and scatter over the apple mixture.
5. Set to bake for 40 minutes at 350 f. Place the baking dish in the preheated oven after five minutes.
6. Enjoy and serve.

86.Apple Cake

Total time: 35 min

Prep time: 15 min

Cook time: 20 min

Yield: 12 serving

Ingredients:

- 2 cups apples, peeled and chopped
- 1/4 cup sugar
- 1/4 cup butter, melted
- 12 oz. apple juice
- 3 cups all-purpose flour
- 3 tsp. baking powder
- 1 1/2 tbsp. ground cinnamon
- 1 tsp. salt

Directions:

1. Place the Cuisinart oven in place 1. with the rack.
2. Mix the rice, salt, sugar, cinnamon, and baking powder together in a big dish.
3. Mix until well mixed, add melted butter and apple juice and mix.

4. Attach apples and fold thoroughly.

5. Pour the batter into the baking bowl, which is greased.

6. Set for 45 minutes to bake at 350 f. Place the baking dish in the preheated oven after five minutes.

7. Enjoy and serve.

87.Almond Cranberry Muffins

Total time: 35 min

Prep time: 15 min

Cook time: 20 min

Yield: 6 serving

Ingredients:

- 2 eggs
- 1 tsp. vanilla
- 1/4 cup sour cream
- 1/2 cup cranberries
- 1 1/2 cups almond flour
- 1/4 tsp. cinnamon
- 1 tsp. baking powder
- 1/4 cup swerve
- Pinch of salt

Directions:

1. Place the Cuisinart oven in place 1. with the rack.

2. Set aside and line 6-cups of a muffin tin with cupcake liners.

3. Put the sour cream, vanilla, and eggs in a cup.

4. Attach the remaining ingredients and beat until smooth, save for the cranberries.

5. Remove cranberries and fold thoroughly.

6. Load the batter into the muffin tin that has been packed.

7. Set for 30 minutes to bake at 325 f. Place the muffin tin in the preheated oven for 5 minutes.

8. Enjoy and serve.

88.Vanilla Butter Cake

Total time: 30 min

Prep time: 10 min

Cook time: 20 min

Yield: 8 serving

Ingredients:

- 1 egg, beaten
- 1/2 tsp. vanilla
- 3/4 cup sugar
- 1 cup all-purpose flour
- 1/2 cup butter, softened

Directions:

1. Place the cuisine-style oven with the rack in place 1.

2. Mix the sugar and butter together in a mixing cup.

3. Apply the egg, rice, and vanilla and whisk until mixed together.

4. Pour in the greased baking dish with the batter.

5. Set for 35 minutes to bake at 350 f. Place the baking sheet in the preheated oven after five minutes.

6. Cut and eat.

89.Coconut Butter Apple Bars

Total time: 40 min

Prep time: 10 min

Cook time: 30 min

Yield: 8 serving

Ingredients:

- 1 tbsp. ground flax seed

- 1/4 cup coconut butter, softened
- 1 cup pecans
- 1 cup of water
- 1/4 cup dried apples
- 1 1/2 tsp. baking powder
- 1 1/2 tsp. cinnamon
- 1 tsp. vanilla
- 2 tbsp. swerve

Directions:

1. Place the cuisine-style oven with the rack in place 1.
2. In the blender, add all of the ingredients and blend until smooth.
3. Pour the mixed mixture into the baking dish with oil.
4. Set to bake for 50 minutes at 350 f. Place the baking sheet in the preheated oven after five minutes.
5. Cut and eat.

90.Easy Blueberry Muffins

Total time: 40 min

Prep time: 10 min

Cook time: 30 min

Yield: 8 serving

Ingredients:

- o   oz. plain yogurt
- ½ cup fresh blueberries
- 2 tsp. baking powder, gluten-free
- ¼ cup swerve
- 2 ½ cups almond flour
- ½ tsp. vanilla
- 3 eggs

- Pinch of salt

Directions:

1. Place the Cuisinart oven in place 1. with the rack.
2. Set aside and line 6-cups of a muffin tin with cupcake liners.
3. Mix the egg, yogurt, vanilla, and salt in a bowl until smooth.
4. Add the flour, swerve and baking powder, and mix until smooth again.
5. Add the blueberries and blend well with them.
6. Load the batter into the muffin tin that has been packed.
7. Placed to bake for 35 minutes at 325 f. Place the muffin tin in the preheated oven for 5 minutes.
8. Enjoy and serve.

91.Tasty Almond Macaroons

Total time: 20 min

Prep time: 10 min

Cook time: 10 min

Yield: 12 serving

Ingredients:

- 2 egg whites
- 10 oz. almonds, sliced
- 1/2 tsp. vanilla extract
- 3/4 cup Splenda

Directions:

1. Place the Cuisinart oven in place 1. with the rack.
2. Beat the egg whites in a bowl until foamy, then add the Splenda and vanilla and mix until low.
3. Apply the egg mixture to the almonds and fold softly.
4. Slip the mixture into the parchment-lined baking pan using a spoon.
5. Set for 15 minutes to bake at 350 f. Place the baking pan in the preheated oven after five minutes.

6. Enjoy and serve.

92.Moist Baked Donuts

Total time: 20 min

Prep time: 10 min

Cook time: 10 min

Yield: 12 serving

Ingredients:

- 2 eggs
- 3/4 cup sugar
- 1/2 cup buttermilk
- 1/4 cup vegetable oil
- 1 cup all-purpose flour
- 1/2 tsp. vanilla
- 1 tsp. baking powder
- 1/2 tsp. salt

Directions:

1. Place the Cuisinart oven in place 1. with the rack.
2. Spray the donut pan and set it aside with the cooking spray.
3. Mix the oil, vanilla, baking powder, sugar, eggs, buttermilk, and salt together in a bowl until well mixed.
4. Stir in the flour and blend until the mixture is tender.
5. Load the batter into the donut pan that has been packed.
6. Set for 20 minutes to bake at 350 f. Place the donut pans in the preheated oven after five minutes.
7. Enjoy and serve.

93.Eggless Brownies

Total time: 40 min

Prep time: 10 min

Cook time: 30 min

Yield: 12 serving

Ingredients:

- 1/4 cup walnuts, chopped
- 1/3 cup cocoa powder
- 2 tsp. baking powder
- 1 cup of sugar
- 1 cup all-purpose flour
- 1/2 cup chocolate chips
- 2 tsp. vanilla
- 1 tbsp. milk
- 3/4 cup yogurt
- 1/2 cup butter, melted
- 1/4 tsp. salt

Directions:

1. Place the cuisine-style oven with the rack in place 1.
2. Sift the rice, chocolate powder, baking powder and salt into a large mixing cup. Mix and put aside well.
3. Add the sugar, vanilla, cream, and yogurt to another dish, and whisk until well mixed.
4. Apply the flour mixture to the mixture of butter and combine until just blended.
5. Fold in some chocolate chips and walnuts.
6. Pour the batter into a baking dish that has been packed.
7. Set to bake for 45 minutes at 350 f. Place the baking sheet in the preheated oven after five minutes.
8. Cut and eat.

94.Vanilla Banana Brownies

Total time: 40 min

Prep time: 10 min

Cook time: 30 min

Yield: 12 serving

Ingredients:

- 1 egg
- 1 cup all-purpose flour
- 4 oz. white chocolate
- 1/4 cup butter
- 1 tsp. vanilla extract
- 1/2 cup granulated sugar
- 2 medium bananas, mashed
- 1/4 tsp. salt

Directions:

1. Place the cuisine-style oven with the rack in place 1.
2. In a microwave-safe mug, add white chocolate and butter, and microwave for 30 seconds. Stir until it melts.
3. Send sugar a stir. Add mashed bananas, vanilla, eggs, and salt and combine until mixed together.
4. Attach rice, then blend until just blended together.
5. Pour in the greased baking dish with the batter.
6. Placed to bake for 25 minutes at 350 f. Place the baking sheet in the preheated oven after five minutes.
7. Cut and eat.

95.Choco Cookies

Total time: 20 min

Prep time: 10 min

Cook time: 10 min

Yield: 12 serving

Ingredients:

- 3 egg whites
- 3/4 cup cocoa powder, unsweetened
- 1 3/4 cup confectioner sugar
- 1 1/2 tsp. vanilla

Directions:

1. Place the Cuisinart oven in place 1. with the rack.
2. Whip the egg whites in a mixing bowl until the soft peaks are fluffy. Add the chocolate, cinnamon, and vanilla slowly.
3. Drop the teaspoonful into 32 tiny cookies on a parchment-lined baking pan.
4. Set for 8 minutes to bake at 350 f. Place the baking pan in the preheated oven after five minutes.
5. Enjoy and serve.

96.Chocolate Chip Cookies

Total time: 20 min

Prep time: 10 min

Cook time: 10 min

Yield: 30 serving

Ingredients:

- 1 egg
- 2/3 cup sugar
- 1 tsp. vanilla
- 1 cup butter, softened
- 12 oz. chocolate chips
- 2 cups self-rising flour
- 1/2 cup brown sugar

Directions:

1. Place the Cuisinart oven in place 1. with the rack.

2. In a broad mixing cup, add the sugar, vanilla, and egg and beat until mixed.

3. Apply the brown sugar and sugar and mix until smooth.

4. Add the flour slowly and stir until just mixed.

5. Fold the chocolate chips together.

6. Spoon the cookie dough balls into a baking tray lined with parchment.

7. Set for 15 minutes to bake at 375 f. Place the baking pan in the preheated oven after five minutes.

8. Enjoy and serve.

97.Oatmeal Cake

Total time: 40 min

Prep time: 10 min

Cook time: 30 min

Yield: 8 serving

Ingredients:

- 2 eggs, beaten
- 1 tbsp. cocoa powder
- 1/2 tsp. salt
- 1 tsp. baking soda
- 1/2 cup butter, softened
- 1 cup granulated sugar
- 1 cup brown sugar
- 1 3/4 cups flour
- 1 cup quick oats
- 3/4 cup mix nuts, chopped
- 2 cups chocolate chips
- 1 3/4 cup boiling water

Directions:

1. Place the cuisine-style oven with the rack in place 1.

2. Combine the boiling water in a large bowl with the oats.

3. Stir in the butter and sugar before the butter has melted.

4. Combine the rice, baking soda, cinnamon, cocoa powder, 1 cup of chocolate chips, half the diced nuts, and the egg. Mix once combined.

5. Sprinkle the remaining nuts and chocolate chips over the top of the cake batter and add the batter into the greased cake tin.

6. Set to bake for 45 minutes at 350 f. Place the baking sheet in the preheated oven after five minutes.

7. Cut and eat.

98. Delicious Banana Cake

Total time: 50 min

Prep time: 10 min

Cook time: 40 min

Yield: 8 serving

Ingredients:

- 2 large eggs, beaten
- 1 tsp. baking powder
- 1 1/2 cup sugar, granulated
- 1 tsp. vanilla extract
- 1/2 cup butter
- 1 cup milk
- 2 cups all-purpose flour
- 2 bananas, mashed
- 1 tsp. baking soda

Directions:

1. Place the cuisine-style oven with the rack in place 1.

2. Beat the sugar and butter together in a mixing bowl until smooth. Beaten eggs are inserted to blend properly.

3. Apply to the mixture the milk, vanilla extract, baking soda, baking powder, flour, and mashed bananas, and beat for 2 minutes. Mix thoroughly.

4. Pour in the greased baking dish with the batter.

5. Set to bake for 45 minutes at 350 f. Place the baking sheet in the preheated oven after five minutes.

6. Slice and eat.

99.Chocolate Cake

Total time: 50 min

Prep time: 10 min

Cook time: 40 min

Yield: 8 serving

Ingredients:

- 1/2 cup warm water
- 2 3/4 cups flour
- 1 cup buttermilk
- 1 cup shortening
- 1 cup sugar, granulated
- 1 cup brown sugar
- 2 large eggs
- 1/2 cup cocoa powder
- 1 tsp. baking soda

Directions:

1. Place the cuisine-style oven with the rack in place 1.

2. Beat together powdered sugar, granulated sugar and shortening until smooth in a large mixing cup.

3. Mix well with the eggs, cocoa powder, rice, and buttermilk when combined.

4. In warm water, dissolve the soda and stir into the batter.

5. Pour in the greased baking dish with the batter.

6. Set for 35 minutes to bake at 350 f. Place the baking sheet in the preheated oven after five minutes.

7. Slice and eat.

100.Almond Blueberry Bars

Total time: 60 min

Prep time: 10 min

Cook time: 40 min

Yield: 8 serving

Ingredients:

- 1/4 cup blueberries
- 3 tbsp. coconut oil
- 2 tbsp. coconut flour
- 1/2 cup almond flour
- 3 tbsp. water
- 1 tbsp. chia seeds
- 1 tsp. vanilla
- 1 tsp. fresh lemon juice
- 2 tbsp. erythritol
- 1/4 cup almonds, sliced
- 1/4 cup coconut flakes

Directions:

1. Place the Cuisinart oven with the rack in place 1.

2. Line a baking dish and set it aside with parchment paper.

3. Mix the water and the chia seeds together in a shallow cup. Put back aside.

4. In a tub, mix all of the ingredients together. Attach a blend of chia and whisk well.

5. Pour the mixture into the baking dish prepared and spread uniformly.

6. Set to bake for 55 minutes, at 300 f. Place the baking dish in the preheated oven after five minutes.

7. Slice and eat.

Conclusion

What is so unique about air frying, though? In a fraction of the time, the air fryer will replace your refrigerator, your fridge, your deep fryer, and your dehydrator, and cook tasty meals uniformly. The air fryer is a game changer if you're trying to supply your family with nutritious meals, just don't have a lot of time. This book is a compilation of 100 amazing and palatable air fryer recipes that you must give a try.

The Essential Air Fryer Cookbook

The Ultimate Air Fryer Cookbook with Quck, Easy and Affordable Recipe

By Marisa Smith

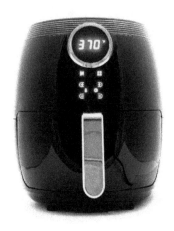

Respective authors own all copyrights not held by the publisher.

The information herein is offered for informational purposes solely and is universal as such. The presentation of the information is without a contract or any type of guarantee assurance.

The trademarks that are used are without any consent, and the publication of the trademark is without permission or backing by the trademark owner. All trademarks and brands within this book are for clarifying purposes only and are owned by the owners themselves, not affiliated with this document.

Introduction

The air fryer raises the amount of heat so that the food gets crispy quicker and faster. Less oil is used for the air fryer, and individuals are happier. In the outer rings and not inside the food, the oils used for cooking French fries or other fried classics. The concept is much better for energy consumption than a traditional fryer. There aren't any open fires or boiling oil pans. You can cook your favorite family meals much easily at home using your air fryer.

Air Fryer Recipes

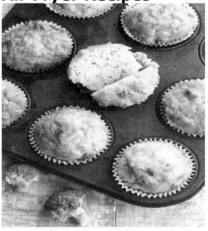

1.Parmesan Muffins

Total time: 20 min

Prep time: 10 min

Cook time: 10 min

Yield: 4 servings

Ingredients:

- 3 oz. Almond milk
- 4 oz. White flour
- 2 oz. Parmesan cheese, grated
- 2 eggs
- 2 tbsp. Olive oil
- 1 tbsp. Baking powder
- A splash of Worcestershire sauce

Directions:

1. Mix the eggs in a bowl with 1 tbsp. Gas, milk, baking powder, flour, and parmesan and Worcestershire sauce; blend well.

2. With the remaining 1 tbsp., grease a muffin pan that suits your air fryer. Divide the cheesy mix equally with the oil and put the pan in the air fryer.

3. Cook for 15 minutes at 320°f. Enjoy

2.Angel Food Cake

Total time: 40 min

Prep time: 15 min

Cook time: 25 min

Yield: 12 servings

Ingredients:

- ¼ cup butter, melted
- 1 cup powdered erythritol
- 1 teaspoon strawberry extract
- 12 egg whites
- 2 teaspoons cream of tartar
- A pinch of salt

Directions:

1. For 5 minutes, preheat the air fryer.

2. Combine the egg whites and the tartar cream.

3. Using a hand mixer and whisk until fluffy and white.

4. Except for the butter, add the rest of the ingredients and whisk for another minute.

5. Pour it into a bowl for baking.

6. Place in a basket of air fryers and cook at 4000f for 30 minutes or if a toothpick inserted in the middle comes out clean.

7. Drizzle until cooled with melted butter.

4. Pumpkin Muffins

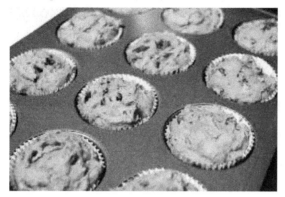

Total time: 35 min

Prep time: 10 min

Cook time: 25min

Yield: 10 serving

Ingredients:

- ¼ cup of butter
- ¾ cup of pumpkin puree
- 2 tablespoons of flaxseed meal
- ¼ cup of flour
- ½ cup of sugar
- ½ teaspoon of nutmeg, ground
- 1 teaspoon of cinnamon powder
- ½ teaspoon of baking soda
- 1 egg
- ½ teaspoon of baking powder

Directions:

1. In a cup, mix the butter, pumpkin puree and egg, then blend properly.

2. Flaxseed meal, flour, sugar, baking soda, baking powder, nutmeg, and cinnamon are mixed well and added.

3. Place this in a fryer at 350 ° F in a muffin pan that matches your fryer, and bake for 15 minutes.

4. Serve as a breakfast for frozen muffins.

4. Zucchini Chips

Total time: 35 min

Prep time: 10 min

Cook time: 25min

Yield: 10 serving

Ingredients:

- 3 zucchinis, thinly sliced
- Salt and black pepper to the taste
- 2 tablespoons of olive oil
- 2 tablespoons of balsamic vinegar

Directions:

1. Mix oil and vinegar, salt and pepper in a cup, then whisk well.

2. Add the zucchini strips, mix well to cover, place in the Air Fryer and cook for 1 hour at 200° F.

3. Serve frozen corvette chips as a snack.

5. Beef Jerky Snack

Total time: 1 hour30 min

Prep time: 30 min

Cook time: 1 hour

Yield: 6 serving

Ingredients:

- 2 cups of soy sauce
- ½ cup of Worcestershire sauce
- 2 tablespoons of black peppercorns
- 2 tablespoons of black pepper
- 2 pounds of beef round, sliced

Directions:

1. In a mug, blend and whisk well the soy sauce with black peppercorns, black pepper, and Worcestershire sauce.

2. Attach slices of beef, swirl to coat, and place in the fridge for 6 hours.

3. Put the beef rounds into your Air Fryer and cook them for 1 hour and 30 minutes at 370° F.

4. Switch to a bowl and eat it cool.

6. Honey Party Wings

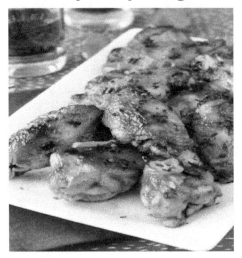

Total time: 30 min

Prep time: 15min

Cook time: 15 min

Yield: 6 serving

Ingredients:

- 16 chicken wings, halved
- 2 tablespoons of soy sauce
- 2 tablespoons of honey
- Salt and black pepper to the taste
- 2 tablespoons of lime juice

Directions:

1. Mix the chicken wings in a bowl of soy sauce, sugar, salt, pepper, and lime juice, mix well, and hold for 1 hour in the refrigerator.

2. Switch the chicken wings to the Air Fryer and cook them for 12 minutes at 360° F, slicing them in half.

3. Put them up on a tray and serve as an appetizer.

7. Salmon Party Patties

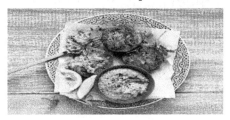

Total time: 30 min

Prep time: 15min

Cook time: 15 min

Yield: 6 serving

Ingredients:

- 3 big potatoes, boiled, drained, and mashed
- 1 big salmon fillet, skinless, boneless
- 2 tablespoons of parsley, chopped
- 2 tablespoon of dill, chopped
- Salt and black pepper to the taste
- 1 egg
- 2 tablespoons of bread crumbs
- Cooking spray

Directions:

1. Place the salmon in the basket of your air fryer and cook at 360 ° F for 10 minutes.
2. Move the salmon to a cutting board, cool it down, place it in a bowl, and flake it.
3. Use this combination to Mix mashed potatoes, salt, pepper, dill, parsley, egg, and bread crumbs, stir well, and form eight patties.

4. Place the salmon patties in the basket of your Air Fryer, spray them with cooking oil, cook for 12 minutes at 360 ° F, turn them halfway, move them to a dish and serve as an appetizer.

8. Banana Chips

Total time: 30 min

Prep time: 15min

Cook time: 15 min

Yield: 6 serving

Ingredients:

- 4 bananas, peeled and sliced
- A pinch of salt
- ½ teaspoon of turmeric powder
- ½ teaspoon of chat masala
- 1 teaspoon of olive oil

Directions:

1. In a bowl, mix banana slices with salt, turmeric, chat masala, and oil, toss and leave aside for 10 minutes.

2. Transfer banana slices to your preheated Air Fryer at 360° F and cook them for 15 minutes, flipping them once.

3. Serve as a snack.

9. Spring Rolls

Total time: 30 min

Prep time: 15min

Cook time: 15 min

Yield: 6 serving

Ingredients:

- 2 cups of green cabbage, shredded
- 2 yellow onions, chopped
- 1 carrot, grated
- ½ chili pepper, minced
- 1 tablespoon of ginger, grated
- 3 garlic cloves, minced
- 1 teaspoon of sugar
- Salt and black pepper to the taste
- 1 teaspoon of soy sauce
- 2 tablespoons of olive oil
- 10 spring roll sheets
- 2 tablespoons of cornflour
- 2 tablespoons of water

Directions:

1. Heat a skillet over medium heat with the oil, add cabbage, onions, carrots, chili pepper, ginger, garlic, sugar, salt, pepper, and soy sauce, mix well, cook for 2-3 minutes, heat off and cool off.

2. Break spring roll sheets into squares, divide and roll cabbage mix on top.

3. Mix cornflour with water in a bowl, stir well and use this mix to seal spring rolls.

4. Put spring rolls in the basket of your Air Fryer, and cook them for 10 minutes at 360° F.

5. Flip the rollover and simmer for another 10 minutes.

6. Set aside on a plate and serve as an appetizer.

10. Crispy Radish Chips

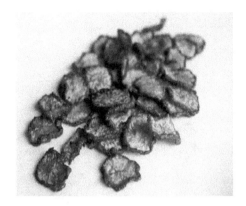

Total time: 25 min

Prep time: 10min

Cook time: 15 min

Yield: 6 serving

Ingredients:

- Cooking spray
- 15 radishes, sliced
- Salt and black pepper to the taste
- 1 tablespoon of chives, chopped

Directions:

1. Arrange radish slices in your Air Fryer's basket, spray them with cooking oil, season with salt and black pepper to the taste, cook them at 350° F for 10 minutes, flipping them halfway, transfer to bowls and serve with chives sprinkled on top.

11. Crab Sticks

Total time: 12 min

Prep time: 2min

Cook time: 10min

Yield: 6 serving

Ingredients:

- 10 crabsticks, halved
- 2 teaspoons of sesame oil
- 2 teaspoons of Cajun seasoning

Directions:

1. Place the crab sticks in a pan, add the sesame oil and the Cajun seasoning, shake, put them in your Air Fryer basket and cook at 350 ° F for 12 minutes. Place it on a tray and eat it as an appetizer.

12. Air Fried Dill Pickles

Total time: 25 min

Prep time: 15min

Cook time: 10min

Yield: 6 serving

Ingredients:

- 16 ounces jarred dill pickles, cut into wedges and pat dry
- ½ cup of white flour
- 1 egg
- ¼ cup of milk
- ½ teaspoon of garlic powder
- ½ teaspoon of sweet paprika
- Cooking spray
- ¼ cup of ranch sauce

Directions:

2. Combine the milk with the egg in a cup and whisk well.
3. Mix the flour with the cinnamon, garlic powder, and paprika in a second bowl and whisk as well.

4. Dip the pickles in the flour, then put them in the egg mixture, then put them back in the flour, and put them in the Air Fryer.

5. Grease with cooking oil, cook the pickle wedges for 5 minutes at 400 ° F, move to a bowl, and serve on the side with ranch sauce.

13. Chickpeas Snack

Total time: 25 min

Prep time: 15min

Cook time: 10min

Yield: 4 serving

Ingredients:

- 15 ounces of canned chickpeas, drained
- ½ teaspoon of cumin, ground
- 1 tablespoon of olive oil
- 1 teaspoon of smoked paprika
- Salt and black pepper to the taste

Directions:

1. Mix the chickpeas with oil, cumin, paprika, salt, and pepper in a dish, mix to cover, put them in the basket of your fryer and cook for 10 minutes at 390° F.

2. Serve as a snack and break into bowls.

14. Beef Short Ribs

Preparation time: 10 minutes

Cooking time: 35 minutes

Servings: 4

Ingredients:

- 1 2/3 lbs. Short ribs

- Salt and black pepper, to taste
- 1 teaspoon grated garlic
- 1/2 teaspoon salt
- 1 teaspoon cumin seeds
- ¼ cup panko crumbs
- 1 teaspoon ground cumin
- 1 teaspoon avocado oil
- ½ teaspoon orange zest
- 1 egg, beaten

Directions:

1. Place a baking tray with the beef ribs and pour the whisked egg on top.

2. In a bowl, whisk the remainder of the crusting ingredients and brush over the meat.

3. Click the air fry oven's "power button" and change the dial to pick the mode for "air fry."

4. To adjust the cooking time to 35 minutes, press the time button and change the dial once again.

5. Now press the temperature button and set the heat at 350 degrees f, and rotate the dial.

6. Position the beef baking tray in the oven until heated up, and close the lid.

7 Serve warm.

15. Tarragon Beef Shanks
Preparation time: 10 minutes

Cooking time: 1hr 30 minutes

Servings: 6

Ingredients:

- 2 tablespoons olive oil
- 2 lbs. Beef shank
- Salt and black pepper to taste
- 1 onion, diced
- 2 stalks celery, diced
- 1 cup marsala wine
- 2 tablespoons dried tarragon

Directions:

1. In a baking pan, put the beef shanks.

2. In a bowl, mix together the remaining ingredients and spill over the shanks.

3. Place these shanks in the basket of an air fryer.

4. Click the air fry oven's "power button" and change the dial to pick the mode for "air fry."

5. To set the cooking time to 1 hr. 30 minutes, click the time button and change the dial again.

6. Now press the temp button and set the heat at 400 degrees f, and rotate the dial.

7. Place the air fryer basket in the oven until preheated and close the lid.

8. Serve it warm.

16. Garlic Braised Ribs

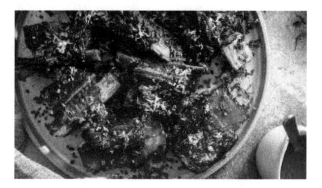

Preparation time: 10 minutes

Cooking time: 1hr 30 minutes

Servings: 10

Ingredients:

- 2 tablespoons vegetable oil
- 5 lbs. Bone-in short ribs
- Salt and black pepper
- 2 heads garlic, halved
- 1 medium onion, chopped
- 4 ribs celery, chopped
- 2 medium carrots, chopped
- 3 tablespoons tomato paste
- ¼ cup dry red wine
- ¼ cup beef stock
- 4 sprigs thyme
- 1 cup parsley, chopped
- ½ cup chives, chopped

- 1 tablespoon lemon zest, grated

Directions:

1. Then toss all this in a large bowl and add the short ribs.

2. To soak the ribs, mix well and marinate for 30 minutes.

3. To the baking pan, shift the soaked ribs and apply the marinade around them.

4. Press the Air Fry Oven control button and change the dial to activate the bake mode.

5. To set the cooking time to 1 hr. 30 minutes, press the time button and change the knob again.

6. Now press the temperature button and set the heat at 400 degrees f, and turn the dial.

7. Place the rib tray in the oven until preheated and close the lid.

8. Serve it warm.

17. BBQ Beef Roast

Preparation time: 10 minutes

Cooking time: 15 minutes

Servings: 4

Ingredients:

- 1lb. Beef roast
- ½ cup bbq sauce

Directions:

1. The beef roast with bbq sauce is completely polished.

2. Place the saucy roast in the basket of an air fryer.

3. Press the air fry oven's "power button" and turn the dial to choose the mode for "air fry."

4. To set the preparation temperature to 15 minutes, press the time button and switch the dial once again.

5. Now push the temperature button to set the temperature at 390 degrees f and turn the dial.

6. Place the air fryer bowl in the oven until preheated and close the lid.

7. When cooked, turn the roast halfway through, then start cooking.

8. Serve it warm.

18. Rosemary Beef Roast
Preparation time: 10 minutes

Cooking time: 15 minutes

Servings: 4

Ingredients:
- 2 lb. Beef roast
- 1 tablespoon olive oil
- 1 medium onion
- 1 teaspoon salt
- 2 teaspoon rosemary and thyme

Directions:
1. Place the beef roast in the basket of an air fryer.

2. Use olive oil, salt, rosemary, thyme, and onion to rub.

3. Press the air fry oven's "power button" and switch the dial to choose the mode for "air fry."

4. To set the cooking time to 15 minutes, click the time button and change the dial once again.

5. Now, push the temperature key to set the temperature at 390 degrees f and turn the dial.

6. Place the air fryer basket in the oven until preheated and close the lid.

7. When cooked, turn the roast halfway through, then start cooking.

8. Serve it warm.

19. Beef Pesto Bake

Preparation time: 10 minutes

Cooking time: 35 minutes

Servings: 6

Ingredients:

- 25 oz. Potatoes, boiled
- 14 oz. Beef mince
- 23 oz. Jar tomato pasta
- 12 oz. Pesto
- 1 tablespoon olive oil

Directions:

1. In a bowl, mash the potatoes and stir in some pesto.

2. In a frying pan, sauté the beef with olive oil once golden.

3. Layer a tomato pasta sauce casserole dish with it.

4. Top that with beef mince sauce.

5. In an even layer, scatter the green pesto potato mash over the meat.

6. Press the Air Fry Oven control button and switch the key to activate the bake mode.

7. To set the cooking time to 35 minutes, press the time button and change the dial once again.

8. Now, push the temp key to level the temperature at 350 degrees f and rotate the dial.

9. Place the casserole dish in the oven until heated up, and close the lid.

10. Serve it warm.

20. Crusted Beef Ribs
Preparation time: 10 minutes

Cooking time: 1hr 40 minutes

Servings: 8

Ingredients:

- 8 beef short ribs, trimmed
- 1/4 cup plain flour
- 1 tablespoon olive oil
- 1 large brown onion, chopped
- 2 garlic cloves, crushed
- 3 medium carrots, peeled and diced
- 2 tablespoons tomato paste
- 2 1/2 cups beef stock
- 2 dried bay leaves
- 1 cup frozen peas
- 3 cups potato gems

Directions:

1. Dust the flour on the ribs of the beef and sear in a pan layered with olive oil.

2. Sear 4 minutes per side of the beef ribs.

3. Shift the ribs to a tray for baking.

4. Add garlic, onion, and carrot to the same pan.

5. Include the tomato paste, stock, and all other ingredients, and sauté for 5 minutes.

6. Cook for four minutes and then add the sauce over the ribs.

7. Press the Air Fry Oven control button and switch the dial to activate the bake mode.

8. To adjust the cooking time to 1 hr. 30 minutes, click the time button and change the knob again.

9. Now push the temp key to set the temperature at 350 degrees f and turn the dial.

10. Place the baking pan in the oven until heated up and close its lid.

11. Serve it warm.

21. Beef Potato Meatballs

Preparation time: 10 minutes

Cooking time: 20 minutes

Servings: 4

Ingredients:

- ½ lb. Minced beef
- 1 tabs parsley chopped
- 2 teaspoon curry powder
- 1 pinch salt and black pepper
- 1 lb. Potato cooked, mashed
- 1 oz. Cheese grated
- 1 ½ oz. Potato chips crushed

Directions:

1. Comb the beef properly in a bowl with the potato and all other ingredients.

2. Form small meatballs out of this combination, then put them in the basket of the air fryer.

3. Press the air fry oven's "power button" and switch the dial to choose the mode for "air fry."

4. To set the cooking time to 20 minutes, click the time button and change the dial once again.

5. Then push the temp button to set the temp at 350 degrees f and rotate the dial.

6. Once heated up, put the basket of meatballs in the oven and close the lid.

7. Once cooked halfway thru, flip the meatballs.

8. Serve it warm.

22. Meatball Bake

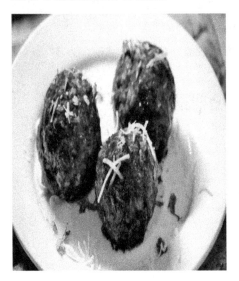

Preparation time: 10 minutes

Cooking time: 35 minutes

Servings: 6

Ingredients:

- 2 tablespoons olive oil
- 2 lbs. Ground beef
- 1 cup ricotta cheese
- 2 large eggs
- 1/2 cup bread crumbs
- 1/4 cup chopped fresh parsley
- 1 tablespoon oregano, chopped
- 2 teaspoons salt
- 1/4 teaspoon crushed red pepper flakes
- 1/2 teaspoon ground fennel

- 4 cups tomato sauce
- 1 ½ cup shredded cheddar cheese

Directions:

1. In a bowl, carefully mix the beef with most of the other meatball ingredients.

2. Make little meatballs out of this mixture and placed them in a saucepan.

3. Pour the sauce on top and drizzle the meatballs with the cheese.

4. Press the Air Fry Oven control button and switch the key to pick the bake mode.

5. To adjust the cooking time to 35 minutes, click the time button and change the dial once again.

6. Now press the heat button to set the temperature at 350 degrees f and rotate the dial.

7. Place the meatballs pan in the oven until preheated and close the lid.

8. Serve warm.

23. Teriyaki Meatballs

Preparation time: 10 minutes

Cooking time: 20 minutes

Servings: 6

Ingredients:

- Meatballs:
- 2 lbs. Ground beef mince
- 3/4 cup panko breadcrumbs
- 2 eggs
- 2 scallions or green onions, finely chopped
- 2 cloves garlic, minced

- 2 tablespoons low sodium soy sauce
- 1 tablespoon wine
- Pinch salt and pepper, to taste
- Teriyaki sauce:
- 1 teaspoon sesame oil
- 2 cloves garlic, minced
- 1/3 cup low sodium soy sauce
- 1/4 cup mirin
- 1/4 cup sake
- 1/4 cup brown sugar
- 1/2 cup water
- 1 tablespoon cornstarch
- 2 tablespoons of water
- 1 teaspoon sriracha or more
- Sesame seeds to garnish

Directions:

1. Thoroughly combine the beef with all of the other ingredients for meatballs in a bowl.

2. Make little meatballs out of this combination, then put them in the basket of the air fryer.

3. Press the Air Fry Oven control button and switch the key to activate the bake function.

4. To adjust the cooking time to 20 minutes, press the timer key and change the dial once again.

5. Now tap the temp button to set the level at 350 degrees f and rotate the dial.

6. Once heated up, put the basket of meatballs in the oven and close the lid.

7. When cooked, turn the meatballs halfway through and then start cooking.

8. Meanwhile, whisk the ingredients for the teriyaki sauce into a saucepan.

9. Cook for 5 minutes or so, stirring until it thickens.

10. Over the meatballs, pour this sauce and garnish with sesame seeds.

11. Serve it warm.

24. Three-Cheese Zucchini Boats

Total time: 35 min

Prep time: 10 min

Cook time: 25 min

Yield: 2 servings

Ingredients:

- 2 medium zucchinis
- 1 tablespoon of avocado oil
- 1/4 cup of low-carb, no-sugar-added pasta sauce
- 1/4 cup of full-Fat: ricotta cheese
- 1/4 cup of shredded mozzarella cheese
- 1/4 teaspoon of dried oregano
- 1/4 teaspoon of garlic powder
- 1/2 teaspoon of dried parsley
- 2tablespoons grated vegetarian Parmesan cheese
- 1 zucchini, cut off 1" from the top and bottom.

Directions:

1. 1 Lengthwise, split the zucchini in half and use a spoon to scrape a little bit of the cavity out, making

space for filling. Clean 2 tablespoons of pasta sauce with oil and apply a spoon to each of the cups.

2. 2 In a big saucepan, blend the ricotta, mozzarella, oregano, garlic powder, and parsley together. Spoon the mixture into each zucchini's shell. Place in shells of packed corvettes

3. 3 Configure the temperature to 350 degrees F and change the timer for 20 minutes.

4. 4 To remove from the fryer cup, use tongs or a spatula and keep it carefully. Hard on Parmesan.

25. Portobello Mini Pizzas

Total time: 20 min

Prep time: 5 min

Cook time: 15 min

Yield: 4 servings

Ingredients:

- 2 large portobello mushrooms
- 2 tablespoons of unsalted butter, melted
- 1/2 teaspoon of garlic powder
- 2/3cup of shredded mozzarella cheese
- 4 grape tomatoes, sliced
- 2 leaves of fresh basil, chopped
- 1 tablespoon of balsamic vinegar

Directions:

1. Excavate the mushrooms' interior and leave behind the tops. Put on each cap with butter and sprinkle with the garlic powder.

2. Cover the sliced tomatoes and the mozzarella for each hat. In a 6-inch circular baking pan, position

each mini pizza. Use the Air Fryer to bring the pan into the basket.

3. Set the temperature for a further 10 minutes to 380 ° F and set the timer.

4. Carefully remove the pizzas from the frying basket and garnish them with basil and vinegar.

26. Veggie Quesadilla

Total time: 15 min

Prep time: 5 min

Cook time: 10 min

Yield: 4 servings

Ingredients:

- 1 tablespoon of coconut oil
- 1/2 medium green bell pepper, seeded and chopped
- 1/4 cup of diced red onion
- 1/4 cup chopped of white mushrooms
- 4 flatbread dough tortillas
- 2/3 cup of shredded pepper jack cheese
- 1/2 medium avocado, peeled, pitted, and mashed
- 1/4 cup of full-Fat: sour cream
- 1/4 cup of mild salsa

Directions:

1. In a medium saucepan, heat the coconut oil at low pressure. Before the peppers begin to soften, add the tomato, onion and mushrooms to the skillet and sauté for 3 to 5 minutes.

2. On a working table, place two tortillas and spread half the cheese on each one. Spread the remaining

cheese, top with sautéed onions, and end with two tortillas left. Within the Air Fryer cup, carefully arrange the quesadillas.

3. Adjust the temperature and set a 5-minute timer to 400° F.

4. Flip the quesadillas halfway into the cooking stage. Serve lightly with salsa, avocado and sour cream.

27. Alternative Tortillas

Total time: 25 min

Prep time: 15 min

Cook time: 10 min

Yield: 2 servings

Ingredients:

- 1 cup of broccoli florets
- 1 cup of quartered Brussels sprouts
- 1/2 cup of cauliflower florets
- 1/4 medium white onion, peeled and sliced
- 1/4" thick1/2 medium green bell pepper, seeded and sliced
- 1 tablespoon of coconut oil
- 2 teaspoons of chili powder
- 1/2 teaspoon of garlic powder
- 1/2 teaspoon of cumin

Directions:

1. Mix all the ingredients in a large tub until the vegetables are fully coated and seasoned with oil.

2. Verse the vegetables onto the Air Fryer tray.

3. Set the temperature to 360° F and for 15 minutes, change the timer.

138

4. Shake it two or three times while cooking. Enjoy and serve.

28. Spinach Artichoke Casserole

Total time: 30 min

Prep time: 10 min

Cook time: 25 min

Yield: 2 servings

Ingredients:

- 1 tablespoon of salted butter, melted
- 1/4 cup of diced yellow onion
- 8 ounces of full-Fat: cream cheese, softened
- 1/3 cup of full-Fat: mayonnaise
- 1/3 cup of full-Fat: sour cream
- 1/4 cup of chopped pickled jalapeños
- 2 cups of fresh spinach, chopped
- 2 cups of cauliflower florets, chopped
- 1 cup of artichoke hearts, chopped

Directions:

1. In a large cup, add the butter, onion, cream cheese, mayonnaise and sour cream. Jalapeños, cauliflower, cabbage and artichokes are rolled in.

2. Pour 4 cups of the mixture into a round baking dish. Cover with tape, and drop the Air Fryer in the basket.

3. Set the temperature to 370° F for 15 minutes and change the timer.

4. In order to brown the top, split foil over the last 2 minutes of preparation. Enjoy and serve.

29. Cheesy Boodle Bake

Total time: 20 min

Prep time: 5 min

Cook time: 15 min

Yield: 4 servings

Ingredients:

- 2 tablespoons of salted butter
- 1/4 cup of diced white onion
- 1/2 teaspoon of minced garlic
- 1/2 cup of heavy whipping cream 2 ounces full-Fat: cream cheese
- 1 cup of shredded sharp Cheddar cheese
- 2 medium zucchinis, spiralized

Directions:

1. Melt the butter in a large saucepan over medium heat. Until softening begins, add the onion and sauté for 1-3 minutes. Stir in the garlic and sauté for 30 seconds, then add the cheese and stir in the cream.

2. Take the fire out of the saucepan and stir in the cheddar. Tie the zucchini and blend it with the sauce, then put it in a 4-cup baking dish. Cover the dish with tape, and place it in an Air Fryer basket.

3. Set the temperature to 370° F and set the eight-minute timer.

1. 4 After 6 minutes, cut the foil and let the top brown for the remaining cooking time. Just shake and serve.

30. Greek Stuffed Eggplant

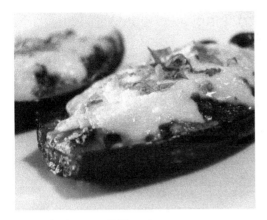

Total time: 35 min

Prep time: 10 min

Cook time: 25 min

Yield: 2 servings

Ingredients:

- 1 large eggplant
- 2 tablespoons of unsalted butter
- 1/4 medium yellow onion, diced
- 1/4 cup of chopped artichoke hearts
- 1 cup of fresh spinach
- 2 tablespoons of diced red bell pepper
- 1/2 cup of crumbled feta

Directions:

1. Break the eggplant lengthwise in half and scrape out the skin, leaving enough space to keep the shell intact. Take the scooped-out eggplant, cut it, and set it aside.

2. Place the butter and onion over low heat in a medium saucepan. Sauté about until the onions tend to soften. 3 to 5 minutes from now. Tie the diced eggplant, lettuce, artichokes, and bell pepper

together. Continue cooking until spinach wilts and peppers soften for 5 minutes. Take the heat off and gently fold in the feta.

3. Insert the filling into each eggplant shell and put it in the Air Fryer basket.

4. Fix the temperature to 320 degrees F and for 20 minutes, set the timer.

5. The eggplant is tender when baked. Enjoy and serve.

31. Roasted Broccoli Salad

Total time: 20 min

Prep time: 5 min

Cook time: 15 min

Yield: 2 servings

Ingredients:

- 3 cups of fresh broccoli florets
- 2 tablespoons of salted butter, melted
- 1/4 cup of sliced almonds
- 1/2 medium lemon

Directions:

1. In a 6' round baking dish, place the broccoli. Scatter the butter over the broccoli, add the almonds, and blend.

2. Set the temperature to 380° F for 7 minutes and change the timer.

3. Pulse halfway into the cooking cycle.

4. On broccoli, zest the lemon and squeeze the juice in a pan while the timer beeps. Shake. Eat hot.

32. Whole Roasted Lemon Cauliflower

Total time: 20 min

Prep time: 5 min

Cook time: 15 min

Yield: 2 servings

Ingredients:

- 1 medium head cauliflower
- 2 tablespoons of salted butter, melted
- 1 medium lemon
- 1/2 medium lemon powder
- 1 teaspoon of dried parsley

Directions:

1. Cut the leaves off the head of the cauliflower and coat them with butter that is melted. Split half the lemon and zest half the cauliflower. Squeeze half the lemon juice with the zest and scatter over the cauliflower.
2. Brush the powder with parsley and garlic. Place the head of the Air Fryer cauliflower in the basket.
3. Fix the temperature to 350 degrees F and for 15 minutes, set the timer.
4. Check the cauliflower every 5 minutes to avoid overcooking. Fork tender is expected to be.
5. Sprinkle another half of the lemon juice over the cauliflower to eat. Serve without hesitation.

33. Cheesy Cauliflower Pizza Crust

Total time: 25 min

Prep time: 5 min

Cook time: 20 min

Yield: 2 servings

Ingredients:

- 1 (12-ounce) steamer bag cauliflower
- 1/2 cup of shredded sharp Cheddar cheese
- 1 large egg
- 2 tablespoons of blanched finely ground almond flour
- 1 teaspoon of Italian blend seasoning

Directions

1. As shown on the package, cook cauliflower. Remove from the bag and place in a cheesecloth or paper towel over water. In a big pan, bring the cauliflower in.

2. Season with a bowl of cheese, honey, almond flour, and Italian cheese and combine well.

3. Cut a piece of parchment with an Air Fryer to fit the bowl. Drive the cauliflower into a 6' diameter circle and place the Air Fryer in the basket.

4. Turn to 360° F and set the 11-minute timer.

5. After 7 minutes, turn the pizza crust over.

34. Apple-Toffee Upside-Down Cake

Total time: 40 min

Prep time: 15 min

Cook time: 25 min

Yield: 9 servings

Ingredients:

- ¼ cup almond butter
- ¼ cup sunflower oil
- ½ cup walnuts, chopped
- ¾ cup + 3 tablespoon coconut sugar

- ¾ cup water
- 1 ½ teaspoon mixed spice
- 1 cup plain flour
- 1 lemon, zest
- 1 teaspoon baking soda
- 1 teaspoon vinegar
- 3 baking apples, cored and sliced

Directions:

1. To 3900f, preheat the air fryer.
2. Melt the almond butter and 3 tablespoons of sugar in a skillet. Over a baking dish that will fit into the air fryer, pour the mixture. On top, arrange the slices of apples. Only set aside.
3. Combine the flour, 3/4 cup sugar, and baking soda in a mixing bowl. Apply the spice blend.
4. Mix the oil, water, vinegar, and lemon zest in another dish. Stir in the walnuts that have been chopped.
5. Combine the wet ingredients: when well mixed, add the dry ingredients.
6. With apple slices, pour over the tin.
7. Bake for 30 minutes, or until the inserted toothpick comes out clean.

35. Blueberry & Lemon Cake

Total time: 40 min

Prep time: 15 min

Cook time: 25 min

Yield: 4 servings

Ingredients:

- 2 eggs
- 1 cup blueberries
- Zest from 1 lemon
- Juice from 1 lemon
- 1 tsp. Vanilla
- Brown sugar for topping (a little sprinkling on top of each muffin-less than a teaspoon)
- 2 1/2 cups self-rising flour
- 1/2 cup monk fruit (or use your preferred sugar)
- 1/2 cup cream
- 1/4 cup avocado oil (any light cooking oil)

Directions:

1. Beat the wet ingredients well in a mixing bowl. Stir in the dry ingredients and blend well.
2. Lightly grease the air-fryer baking pan with cooking oil. Pour the batter in.
3. Cook at 330F for 12 minutes.
4. Let it stand for 5 minutes in an air-fryer.
5. Enjoy and serve.

36. Cherries 'N Almond Flour Bars

Total time: 40 min

Prep time: 15 min

Cook time: 25 min

Yield: 12 servings

Ingredients:

- ¼ cup water
- ½ cup butter softened

- ½ teaspoon salt
- ½ teaspoon vanilla
- 1 ½ cups almond flour
- 1 cup erythritol
- 1 cup fresh cherries, pitted
- 1 tablespoon xanthan gum
- 2 eggs

Directions:

1. Combine the first 6 ingredients in a mixing bowl until the dough shapes.
2. In a baking dish that works in an air fryer, press the dough.
3. Place it in an air fryer and bake at 3750f for 10 minutes.
4. Meanwhile, in a tub, combine the cherries, water, and xanthan gum.
5. Take out the dough and pour the cherry mixture over it.
6. Return to the air-fryer and cook at 3750f for 25 more minutes.

37. Fried Oreos

Total time: 10 min

Prep time: 5 min

Cook time: 5 min

Yield: 8 servings

Ingredients

- 8 Oreo cookies or other brand sandwich cookies
- 1 package of Pillsbury Crescents Rolls (or crescent dough sheet)

- Powdered sugar for dusting

Directions

1. Layout a cutting board or counter with crescent pastry.

2. Push down onto each perforated line using your finger so that one wide sheet shapes.

3. Breakthrough eighths of the dough.

4. In the middle of each of the crescent roll squares, put an Oreo cookie and roll each corner up (see visual above in post).

5. To make sure that it protects the whole Oreo cookie, bunch up the remainder of the crescent roll. Do not stretch too thin on the crescent roll, or it will crack.

6. Preheat the air-fryer for around 2-3 minutes to 320 degrees.

7. Gently put the Air Fried Oreos in an even row within the air fryer so that they do not touch. Cook in batches if you've got a smaller air fryer.

8. Cook the Oreos for 5-6 minutes at 320 degrees, until golden brown on the outside.

9. Remove the Air Fryer Oreos carefully from the air fryer and sprinkle them instantly with powdered sugar if desired.

10. Let the two minutes cool, then enjoy it.

38. Jelly Donuts
Total time: 15 min

Prep time: 5 min

Cook time: 10 min

Yield: 8 servings

Ingredients

- 1 package Pillsbury Grands (Homestyle)
- 1/2 cup seedless raspberry jelly
- 1 tablespoon butter, melted
- 1/2 cup sugar

Directions

1. Preheat the fryer to 320 degrees Celsius.
2. Place the Grand Rolls in one single layer inside the air fryer and cook until golden brown for 5-6 minutes.
3. Set aside and remove the rolls from the air fryer.
4. Place sugar with a flat bottom in a large tub.
5. On both sides of the donut, baste the butter and roll in the sugar to fully coat it. Full with all the donuts left.
6. Pip 1-2 teaspoons of raspberry jelly into each donut using a long cake tip.
7. Enjoy or keeping up to 3 days immediately.

39. Apple Fritters

Total time: 21 min

Prep time: 10 min

Cook time: 6 min

Yield: 8 servings

Ingredients

- 2 apples, cored and diced
- 1 cup all-purpose flour
- 2 tablespoons sugar
- 1 teaspoon baking powder

- 1/2 teaspoon salt
- 1/2 teaspoon ground cinnamon
- 1/4 teaspoon ground nutmeg
- 1/3 cup milk
- 2 tablespoons butter, melted
- 1 egg
- 1/2 teaspoon lemon juice

Cinnamon Glaze

- 1/2 cup confectioners' sugar
- 2 tablespoons milk
- 1/2 teaspoon ground cinnamon
- Pinch of salt

Directions

1. Dice the apples and set them aside in small cubes. If needed, peel them.
2. In a large mixing bowl, add the flour, sugar, baking powder, salt, ground cinnamon, and ground nutmeg and whisk to combine.
3. Mix the milk, butter, egg, and lemon juice in a separate cup.
4. Apply the dry ingredients to the wet ingredients and stir until mixed. Stir in the apples and put the mixture in the refrigerator for about 5 minutes and 2 days (covered).
5. Preheat your 370-degree air fryer.
6. Place a round of parchment on the bottom of the basket and scoop out the 2-tablespoon balls of apple fritters. In an air fryer, put the apple fritters and cook for 6-7 minutes.

7. When cooking, whisk together the candy, sugar, milk, cinnamon, and salt to make the glaze.

8. Remove the apple fritters from the air fryer, position them on a wire rack, and pour the glaze over the top immediately and enjoy.

40. Dessert Fries

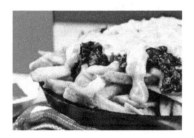

Total time: 20 min

Prep time: 5 min

Cook time: 15 min

Yield: 8 servings

Ingredients

- 2 sweet potatoes
- 1 tablespoon butter, melted
- 1 teaspoon butter, melted and separated from the above
- 2 tablespoons sugar
- 1/2 teaspoon cinnamon

Directions

1. Preheat your 380-degree air fryer.

2. Peel the sweet potatoes and cut them into skinny fries.

3. Using 1 tablespoon of butter to cover the fries.

4. In the preheated air fryer, cook the fries for 15-18 minutes. They can overlap, but more than 1/2 complete shouldn't fill your air fryer.

5. From the air fryer, remove the sweet potato fries and put them in a cup.

6. Coat the remaining butter and add sugar and cinnamon to the mixture. To coat, blend.

7. Immediately enjoy

41. Pumpkin Twists

Total time: 13 min

Prep time: 5 min

Cook time: 6 min

Yield: 8 servings

Ingredients

- 1 can Pillsbury crescent rolls
- 1/8 teaspoon salt
- 3 tablespoons unsalted butter, melted
- 1/2 cup pumpkin puree
- 2 teaspoons pumpkin pie spice

Icing

- 1/2 cup confectionery sugar
- 2 and 1/4 teaspoons milk
- 2 tablespoons melted butter

Directions

1. Mix all the ingredients well in a bowl.

2. Preheat the air fryer at 180 f.

3. Place the baking pan with the batter inside.

4. Bake for 6 minutes

42. Fried Apples

Total time: 13 min

Prep time: 5 min

Cook time: 6 min

Yield: 8 servings

Ingredients

- 3 Granny Smith Apples
- 1 cup flour
- 3 eggs, whisked
- 1 cup graham cracker crumbs
- 1/4 cup sugar
- 1 teaspoon ground cinnamon

Optional

- Caramel sauce for dipping

Directions

1. Preheat your 380-degree air fryer.
2. Cut the apples and remove the core into wedges.
3. Place the flour in the first bowl, the egg in the second bowl, using 3 cups, and mix in the third bowl the graham cracker crumbs, sugar, and cinnamon.
4. In the flour, then the egg, and eventually the graham cracker mixture, dip an apple wedge, making sure to cover the apple as best as possible each time.
5. Repeat with slices of the remaining apple.
6. Place apples in one spaced layer in the air fryer and cook for 5-6 minutes, flipping with one-minute leftover.

7. Remove and enjoy the apples from the Air Fryer! Serve if needed with caramel sauce

43. Air Fryer Smores

Total time: 10 min

Prep time: 2 min

Cook time: 8 min

Yield: 8 servings

Ingredients

- 4 graham crackers broken in half
- 4 large marshmallows
- 1 milk chocolate bar, divided

Directions

1. In the air fryer basket, put four graham cracker halves inside the

2. TRICK: Cut off the bottom of each marshmallow with a tiny slice, and stick it to the graham cracker. During cooking, this will keep it clean.

3. Cook for about 7-8 minutes at 375 degrees, or until the marshmallow is golden brown.

4. Attach Hershey's chocolate to the appropriate amount and top with the other graham cracker.

5. Return for another 2 minutes or before the chocolate starts to melt in the air fryer.

44. Sausage Balls

Total time: 25 min

Prep time: 15min

Cook time: 10min

Yield: 4 serving

Ingredients:

- 4 ounces of sausage meat, ground
- Salt and black pepper to the taste
- 1 teaspoon of sage
- ½ teaspoon of garlic, minced
- 1 small onion, chopped
- 3 tablespoons of breadcrumbs

Directions:

1. In a bowl, mix sausage with salt, pepper, sage, garlic, onion, and breadcrumbs, stir well and shape small balls out of this mix.

2. Put them in your Air Fryer's basket, cook at 360° F for 15minutes, divide into bowls and serve as a snack.

45. Chicken Dip

Total time: 25 min

Prep time: 15min

Cook time: 10min

Yield: 4 serving

Ingredients:

- 3 tablespoons of butter, melted
- 1 cup of yogurt
- 12 ounces of cream cheese
- 2 cups of chicken meat, cooked and shredded
- 2 teaspoons of curry powder
- 4 scallions, chopped
- 6 ounces of Monterey jack cheese, grated
- 1/3 cup of raisins
- ¼ cup of cilantro, chopped

- ½ cup of almonds, sliced
- Salt and black pepper to the taste
- ½ cup of chutney

Directions:

1. In a bowl, mix cream cheese with yogurt and whisk using your mixer.

2. Add curry powder, scallions, chicken meat, raisins, cheese, cilantro, salt, and pepper and stir everything.

3. Spread this into a baking dish that fist your Air Fryer, sprinkle almonds on top, place in your Air Fryer, bake at 300° for 25minutes, divide into bowls, top with chutney, and serve as an appetizer.

46. Sweet Popcorn

Total time: 25 min

Prep time: 15min

Cook time: 10min

Yield: 4 serving

Ingredients:

- 2 tablespoons of corn kernels
- 2 and ½ tablespoons of butter
- 2 ounces of brown sugar

Directions:

1. Place the corn kernels in the pan of your Air Fryer, cook them for 6 minutes at 400° F, move them to a plate, spread them out, and set them aside for now.

2. Heat a casserole over low pressure, add butter, melt it, add sugar, and whisk before dissolving.

3. Add popcorn, throw to cover, heat off and scatter over the tray again.

4. Refrigerate, break into bowls, and serve as a snack.

47. Apple Chips

Total time: 25 min

Prep time: 15min

Cook time: 10min

Yield: 4 serving

Ingredients:

- 1 apple, cored and sliced
- A pinch of salt
- ½ teaspoon of cinnamon powder
- 1 tablespoon of white sugar

Directions:

1. Mix apple slices with salt, sugar, and cinnamon in a cup, swirl, move to the basket from your Air Fryer, cook at 390° F, tossing once for 10 minutes.

2. The apple chips are split into bowls and served as a snack.

48. Bread Sticks

Total time: 25 min

Prep time: 15min

Cook time: 10min

Yield: 4 serving

Ingredients:

- 4 bread slices, each cut into 4 sticks
- 2 eggs
- ¼ cup of milk
- 1 teaspoon of cinnamon powder

- 1 tablespoon of honey
- ¼ cup of brown sugar
- A pinch of nutmeg

Directions:

1. In a cup, add the eggs with the milk, brown sugar, cinnamon, nutmeg, and honey and whisk well.
2. Dip the breadsticks in this mix, place them in your Air Fryer basket, and cook at 360 °F for 10 minutes.
3. Divide the breadsticks into bowls and eat them as a snack.

49. Crispy Shrimp

Total time: 25 min

Prep time: 15min

Cook time: 10min

Yield: 4 serving

Ingredients:

- 12 big shrimp, deveined and peeled
- 2 egg whites
- 1 cup of coconut, shredded
- 1 cup of panko bread crumbs
- 1 cup of white flour
- Salt and black pepper to the taste

Directions:

1. In a bowl, mix panko with coconut and stir.

2. Put flour, salt, and pepper in a second bowl and whisk egg whites in the third one.

3. Dip shrimp in flour, egg whites mix, and coconut, place them all in your Air Fryer's basket, and cook at 350° F for 10 minutes, flipping halfway.

4. Arrange on a platter and serve as an appetizer.

50. Cajun Shrimp Appetizer

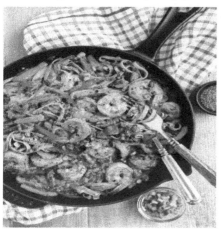

Total time: 15 min

Prep time: 5min

Cook time: 10min

Yield: 2 serving

Ingredients:

- 20 tiger shrimp, peeled and deveined
- Salt and black pepper to the taste
- ½ teaspoon of old bay seasoning
- 1 tablespoon of olive oil
- ¼ teaspoon of smoked paprika

Directions:

1. Mix in the shrimp and the milk, the salt, the pepper, the spice of the old bay, the paprika in the bowl, and mix to cover.

2. Place your Air Fryer shrimp in the basket and cook at 390 ° F for 5 minutes.

3. Put them up on a tray to serve as an appetizer.

51. Crispy Fish Sticks

Total time: 15 min

Prep time: 5min

Cook time: 10min

Yield: 2 serving

Ingredients:

- 4 ounces of bread crumbs
- 4 tablespoons of olive oil
- 1 egg, whisked
- 4 white fish filets, boneless, skinless, and cut into medium sticks
- Salt and black pepper to the taste

Directions:

1. Mix the bread crumbs in a cup with the oil, then whisk well.

2. Place the potato in a second pan, add the salt and pepper and whisk well.

3. Dip the fish stick and bread crumb mix in the egg, place them in your Air Fryer basket, and cook at 360° F for 12 minutes.

4. Place the sticks of fish on a tray and serve as an appetizer.

52. Fish Nuggets

Total time: 15 min

Prep time: 5min

Cook time: 10min

Yield: 2 serving

Ingredients:

- 28 ounces of fish fillets, skinless and cut into medium pieces
- Salt and black pepper to the taste
- 5 tablespoons of flour
- 1 egg, whisked
- 5 tablespoons of water
- 3 ounces of panko bread crumbs
- 1 tablespoon of garlic powder
- 1 tablespoon of smoked paprika
- 4 tablespoons of homemade mayonnaise
- Lemon juice from ½ lemon
- 1 teaspoon of dill, dried
- Cooking spray

Directions:

1. Mix the flour and water in a dish, then mix well.

2. Add potato, pepper, and salt and whisk well.

3. Mix the panko with the garlic powder and paprika in a second dish, then stir well.

4. Sprinkle the pieces of fish in flour and egg mixture and then in panko mixture, put them in the basket of your Air Fryer, spray them with the cooking oil and cook for 12 minutes at 400° F.

5. Meanwhile, blend dill and lemon juice mayo in a bowl, and whisk well.

6. Arrange fish nuggets on a pan, then serve side by side with dill mayo.

53. Shrimp and Chestnut Rolls

Total time: 15 min

Prep time: 5min

Cook time: 10min

Yield: 2 serving

Ingredients:

- ½ pound of already cooked shrimp, chopped
- 8 ounces of water chestnuts, chopped
- ½ pounds of shiitake mushrooms, chopped
- 2 cups of cabbage, chopped
- 2 tablespoons of olive oil
- 1 garlic clove, minced
- 1 teaspoon of ginger, grated
- 3 scallions, chopped
- Salt and black pepper to the taste
- 1 tablespoon of water
- 1 egg yolk
- 6 spring roll wrappers

Directions:

1. Heat the skillet with the oil, add the cabbage, shrimp, chestnuts, mushrooms, garlic, ginger, salt and pepper over medium-high pressure, stir and boil for 2 minutes.
2. Mix the egg and water in a pan and then blend well.
3. Organize roll wrappers on a work surface, slice shrimp and veggie mix into them, seal edges with egg wash, put all of them in your Air Fryer basket, cook 15 minutes at 360 ° F, move to a pan, and serve as an appetizer.

54. Quiche-Stuffed Peppers

Total time: 20 min

Prep time: 5 min

Cook time: 15 min

Yield: 2 serving)

Ingredients:

- 2 medium green bell peppers
- 3 large eggs
- 1/4 cup of full-Fat: ricotta cheese
- 1/4 cup of diced yellow onion
- 1/2 cup of chopped broccoli
- 1/2 cup of shredded medium Cheddar cheese

Directions:

1. Break the tops of the peppers off and use a small knife to remove the white membranes and seeds.
2. In a big saucepan, stir in the eggs and ricotta.
3. Stir in the broccoli and onion. Pour the mixture of vegetables and eggs equally into each pepper. The Cheddar Top. In a 4-cup baking dish, arrange the peppers and placed them in the Air Fryer's basket.
4. Set the temperature for 15 minutes to 350° F and change the timer.
5. The eggs will mainly be solid when fully baked, and the peppers will be tender. Serve without hesitation.

55. Roasted Garlic White Zucchini Rolls

Total time: 40 min

Prep time: 15 min

Cook time: 25 min

Yield: 4 serving)

Ingredients:

- 2 medium zucchinis
- 2 tablespoons of unsalted butter
- 1/4 white onion, peeled and diced
- 1/2 teaspoon of finely minced roasted garlic
- 1/4 cup of heavy cream
- 2 tablespoons of vegetable broth
- 1/8 teaspoon of xanthan gum
- 1/2 cup of full-Fat: ricotta cheese
- 1/4 teaspoon of salt
- 1/2 teaspoon of garlic powder
- 1/4 teaspoon of dried oregano
- 2 cups of spinach, chopped
- 1/2 cup of sliced baby portobello mushrooms
- 3/4 cup of shredded mozzarella cheese, divided

Directions:

1. Break the zucchini lengthwise into long strips using a mandolin or a sharp knife. Place streaks between paper towels to trap moisture. Place yourself aside.

2. Melt the butter in a medium saucepan over a low flame. Add the onion and sauté until it is slightly fragrant. Then add and sauté the garlic for 30 seconds.

3. Add the heavy cream, soup, and xanthan gum to the garnish. Turn off the heat and whisk the mixture until it begins to thicken, for around 3 minutes.

4. In a medium saucepan, add the ricotta, cinnamon, garlic powder, and oregano and mix well. Fold in 1/2 cup mozzarella, onions and spinach.

5. In a 6' round baking pan, add half of the sauce. To arrange the rolls, place two strips of zucchini on a working surface. Spread and roll up 2 teaspoons of ricotta on the slices. Place the seam side down on top of the sauce. For the remaining ingredients, repeat.

1. Scatter with leftover mozzarella, cover with foil, and put in the basket of the fryer. 6. Remaining sauce over the rolls.

6. Set the temperature for 20 minutes to 350 ° F, then set the timer.

7. In the last 5 minutes, cut the foil to brown the cheese. Serve immediately.

56. Spicy Parmesan Artichokes

Total time: 20 min

Prep time: 5 min

Cook time: 15 min

Yield: 4 serving)

Ingredients:

- 2 medium artichokes, trimmed and quartered, center removed
- 2tablespoons of coconut oil
- 1 large egg, beaten
- 1/2 cup of grated vegetarian Parmesan cheese
- 1/4 cup of blanched finely ground almond flour
- 1/2 teaspoon of crushed red pepper flakes

Directions:

1. In a big bowl, toss the artichokes in the coconut oil, then dip each bite into the shell.

2. Whisk the parmesan and almond flour together in a big bowl. Scatter with pepper flakes, tie pieces of artichoke and blend, to cover as fully as possible.

3. Set the temperature to 400 degrees F and for 10 minutes, change the timer.

4. Shake the basket two times before cooking. Serve and enjoy!

57. Zucchini Cauliflower Fritters

Total time: 27 min

Prep time: 5 min

Cook time: 17 min

Yield: 4 serving)

Ingredients:

- 1 (12-ounce) cauliflower steamer bag
- 1 medium zucchini, shredded
- 1/4 cup of almond flour
- 1 large egg
- 1/2 teaspoon of garlic powder
- 1/4 cup of grated vegetarian Parmesan cheese

Directions:

1. In a cheesecloth or paper towel, cook cauliflower according to package instructions and remove excess moisture. Put yourself in a big shower.

2. To remove extra moisture, put the corvettes in a paper towel and pat them down. Apply the cup to the cauliflower. Add remaining products.

3. Break the mixture uniformly, and shape four patties. Push in 1/4'-thick patties. Put each of them in the Air Fryer's basket.

4. Set the temperature to 320 ° F, and for 12 minutes, change the timer.

5. When thoroughly cooked, the fritters should be solid. Give 5 minutes to cool before moving. Serve hot.

58. Basic Spaghetti Squash

Total time: 55 min

Prep time: 25 min

Cook time: 30 min

Yield: 4 serving)

Ingredients:

- 1/2 large spaghetti squash
- 1 tablespoon of coconut oil
- 2 tablespoons of salted butter, melted
- 1/2 teaspoon of garlic powder
- 1teaspoon of dried parsley

Directions:

1. Spaghetti squash rubbed with coconut oil. Brush the butter through and position the side of the skin downwards. Sprinkle with garlic powder and parsley.

2. With the side of the skin down, place the squash in the Air Fryer basket.

3. Adjust the temperature to 350° F and set the timer for 30 minutes.

4. Rotate the squash as the beeps on the timer so that the side of the skin is up and cook for 15 minutes or until tender. Serve and enjoy.

59. Spaghetti Squash Alfredo

Total time: 2: 25in

Prep time: 5 min

Cook time: 20 min

Yield: 4 serving

Ingredients:

- 1/2 large cooked spaghetti squash
- 2 tablespoons of salted butter, melted
- 1/2 cup of low-carb Alfredo sauce
- 1/4 cup of grated vegetarian Parmesan cheese
- 1/2 teaspoon of garlic powder
- 1 teaspoon of dried parsley
- 1/4 teaspoon of ground peppercorn
- 1/2 cup of shredded Italian blend cheese

Directions:

1. To trim spaghetti squash threads from the shell, use a fork. Put the Alfredo sauce in a large, buttered dish. Sprinkle with garlic powder, parmesan, parsley, and peppercorn.
2. Garnish it in a 4-cup oval baking dish with melted cheese. Drop the dish onto an Air Fryer tray.
3. Fix the temperature to 320 degrees F and for 15 minutes, set the timer.
4. It is golden until the cheese is finished, and it explodes. Serve without hesitation.

60. Capers Eggplant Stacks

Total time: 17 min

Prep time: 5 min

Cook time: 12 min

Yield: 4 serving

Ingredients:

- 1 medium eggplant, cut into1/4" slices
- 2 large tomatoes, cut into1/4" slices
- 4ounces of fresh mozzarella cut into1/2-ounce slices
- 2tablespoons of olive oil
- 1/4 cup of fresh basil, sliced

Directions:

1. On the bottom of a 6' round baking dish, place four slices of eggplant. On top of each round eggplant, placed a slice of tomato, then mozzarella, then eggplant.
2. Drizzle with olive oil. Put the dish and cover it with foil in the Air Fryer basket.
3. Set the temperature to 350 ° F and change the 12-minute timer.
4. Once finished, the eggplant will be tender. Garnish it with fresh basil to eat.

61. Crustless Spinach Cheese Pie

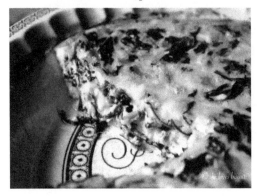

Total time: 25 min

Prep time: 5 min

Cook time: 20 min

Yield: 4 serving

Ingredients:

- 6 large eggs
- 1/4 cup of heavy whipping cream
- 1 cup of frozen chopped spinach, drained
- 1cup of shredded sharp Cheddar cheese
- 1/4 cup of diced yellow onion

Directions:

1. Whisk the eggs in a medium bowl and apply the remaining ingredients to the bowl's milk.
2. Place the Air Fryer in a 6' round baking dish in the basket.
3. Set the temperature to 320 ° F and change the 20-minute timer.
4. The eggs become solid and finely browned when baked.

5. Immediately serve.

94. Broccoli Crust Pizza

Total time: 27 min

Prep time: 10 min

Cook time: 17 min

Yield: 4 serving

Ingredients:

- 3 cups of riced broccoli, steamed and drained well
- 1 large egg
- 1/2 cup of grated vegetarian Parmesan cheese
- 3 tablespoons of low-carb Alfred sauce
- 1/2 cup of shredded mozzarella cheese

Directions:

1. Mix broccoli, egg, and parmesan in a large saucepan.

2. Cut a piece of parchment to match your basket with an Air Fryer. To suit the paper, press out the pizza mixture and work in two lots if necessary. Put the basket into the Air Fryer.

3. Set the temperature to 370° F and change the timer for 5 minutes.

4. The crust should be solid enough to turn as the timer beeps. If not, so add another 2 minutes—crust flip.

5. Finish with mozzarella and Alfredo sauce. Return to the basket with the Air Fryer and cook for 7 minutes or until the cheese is crispy and bubbling. Serve hot and enjoy!

62. Italian Baked Egg and Veggies

Total time: 20 min

Prep time: 5 min

Cook time: 15 min

Yield: 2 serving

Ingredients:

- 2 tablespoons of salted butter
- 1 small zucchini, sliced lengthwise and quartered
- 1/2 medium green bell pepper, seeded and diced
- 1 cup of fresh spinach, chopped
- 1 medium Roma tomato, diced
- 2 large eggs
- 1/4 teaspoon of onion powder
- 1/4 teaspoon of garlic powder
- 1/2 teaspoon of dried basil
- 1/4 teaspoon of dried oregano

Directions:

1. Grease 2 buttered ramekins, each holding 1 tablespoon.
2. In a big bowl, throw the corvettes, bell pepper, spinach, and tomatoes. Put half a ramekin in each and split the mixture into two.
3. On top of each ramekin, split the egg and sprinkle with the onion powder, garlic powder, basil, and oregano. Put the Air Fryer basket back.
4. Fix the temperature for 10 minutes to 330° F and adjust the timer.
5. Immediately serve.

63. BBQ "Pulled" Mushrooms

Total time: 20 min

Prep time: 5 min

Cook time: 15 min

Yield: 2 serving

Ingredients:

- 4 large portobello mushrooms
- 1 tablespoon of salted butter, melted
- 1/4 teaspoon of ground black pepper
- 1teaspoon of chili powder
- 1 teaspoon of paprika
- 1/4 teaspoon of onion powder
- 1/2 cup of low-carb, sugar-free barbecue sauce

Directions:

1. Take the stem off and scoop beneath each mushroom. Using cinnamon, chili powder, paprika, and onion powder to put butter on the caps and dust.

2. Place the mushrooms inside the Air Fryer's basket.

3. Set the temperature to 400° F and set the eight-minute timer.

4. If the timer beeps, remove the mushrooms from the basket and put them on a cutting board or table. With two scissors, please take the mushrooms apart. Build beams.

5. Place the mushroom stems into a 4-cup circular baking dish with the barbecue sauce. Lower the dish into the Air Fryer tray.

6. Set the temperature to 350 degrees F and change the 4-minute timer.

7. Pulse halfway through the cooking cycle. Serve it warm.

64. Air Fryer Churros

Total time: 23 min

Prep time: 15 min

Cook time: 8 min

Yield: 24 servings

Ingredients

- 1/2 cup water
- 1/2 cup milk
- 1/2 cup butter
- 1 Tablespoon granulated sugar
- 1 cup all-purpose flour
- 3 eggs
- 1 teaspoon vanilla

Cinnamon Sugar Coating

- 1 cup granulated sugar
- 1 Tablespoon ground cinnamon

Directions

1. Combine the water, milk, butter and 1 tablespoon of sugar in a medium saucepan. Over medium heat, bring it to a boil, stirring as it heats.
2. Remove the pan from the heat and stir in the flour with a wooden spoon into the saucepan. Stir until it is fully mixed in with the flour.

3. Return the saucepan to heat and stir it for 2 minutes continuously until the dough comes together in a smooth ball.

4. Take the heat off the dough and place the dough in a large mixing bowl.

5. Beat the dough until moist with an electric mixer. This will cool the dough so that when they are inserted, the eggs do not cook. For 3-5 minutes, beat the dough.

6. Whisk the eggs and vanilla extract together in a small cup.

7. In the tub, slowly add the egg mixture to the cooled dough, beating after each addition with the mixer. The sides of the mixing bowl are scraped down and proceed until the eggs are mixed in, and the dough is smooth.

8. Using a plastic pastry bag with a zippered bag with the corner cut off to pipe the churros.

9. Attach the pastry bag to the dough or place it in a plastic bag. Do not cut the corner off while you are using a plastic bag until the dough has been applied.

10. Pipe the dough directly into the basket of the air fryer and cut the end with scissors. I typically make 3-inch churros, but to fit into your air fryer basket, you can change the length as desired. Smaller bits of churro are fun to make as well.

11. Using a master bottle to spray churros with a little bit of oil until all the churros are in the basket.

12. Cook at 380 F for 8-10 minutes or until it is golden brown.

13. Combine the cinnamon sugar mixture in a medium bowl as you cook the churros.

14. Remove the churros from the air fryer and immediately apply to the cinnamon-sugar mixture. Toss them and cover them with cinnamon sugar, and place them to cool on the baking rack.

15. For dipping, serve immediately with chocolate syrup, caramel sauce or Novella.

65. Air Fryer Brownies

Total time: 25 min

Prep time: 5 min

Cook time: 20 min

Yield: 6 servings

Ingredients

- 4 tbsp. Salted Butter
- ¼ cup White Sugar
- ¼ cup Brown Sugar
- ¼ cup Cocoa Powder
- ½ tsp. Vanilla
- 1 Egg
- ¼ cup All Purpose / Plain Flour
- ⅕ cup Chocolate Chips

Optional

- ¼ cup Milk chocolate chunks or chunks of your favorite chocolate bar mixed in for extra chocolate goodness.

Directions

1. Line 2 mini loaf pans or 1 loaf pan of standard size with baking paper.

2. In a microwave-proof dish, put the butter, brown sugar, white sugar and cocoa powder. Microwave in 20-second batches until butter is melted and well mixed, stirring well after each time.

3. To mix through, add vanilla and swirl. Put the bowl aside to allow it to cool slightly for a minute.

4. Mix the egg, add the flour and mix well until mixed. Fold the chocolate chips in (and the optional chocolate chunks if using).

5. Divide the mixture evenly around the mini loaf pans prepared (or only pour into the 1 loaf pan if that's what you're using), and bake for 20-25 minutes in the air fryer on 160C / 320F or until a toothpick inserted comes out with just a few fudgy crumbs attached.☐ Leave the brownie in the loaf pans for 10 minutes to cool, then transfer to a wire rack to cool completely.

66. Domino's Cinnamon Bread Twists

Total time: 25 min

Prep time: 5 min

Cook time: 20 min

Yield: 6 servings

Ingredients

For the Bread Twists Dough

- 1 C (120g) All-Purpose Flour

- 1 tsp. Baking Powder
- 1/4 tsp. Kosher Salt (1/8 tsp. table salt)
- 2/3 C (150g) Fat-Free Greek Yogurt

For Brushing on the Cooked Bread Twists

- 2 Tbsp. (28g) Light Butter*
- 2 Tbsp. (24g) Granulated Sugar*
- 1-2 tsp. Ground Cinnamon, to taste

Directions

1. Before adding the Greek yogurt, combine the flour, baking powder, and salt together. To stir all together, use a fork until a crumbly dough starts to shape. There should be some dry flour left in the tub.

2. On a flat surface, move the crumbly dough and work the dough into one smooth ball of dough. Bring the dough into six bits of 45 grams. Roll the pieces of dough between your palms or form thin lines, about 8 inches long, on the flat surface.

3. To form a ribbon shape, fold one end of each strip over and move to an air fryer basket sprayed with cooking spray. Spray the top with cooking spray and close the lid until all six bread twists are in the basket.

4. Air fried for 15 minutes at 350oF. (Or bake directly on a baking sheet at 375oF for 25-30 minutes.)

5. Microwave the light butter and mix in the granulated sugar and cinnamon at the end of cooking. Brush the cinnamon sugar butter as soon as they come out of the air fryer on top of the bread twists. Serve warm

67. Donuts with Chocolate Glaze

Total time: 10 min

Prep time: 5 min

Cook time: 5 min

Yield: 8 servings

Ingredients

Donuts

- 1 package Grand Flakey Biscuit

Chocolate Glaze Recipe

- 1 cup Powdered Sugar
- 3 1/2 tablespoons Cocoa Powder
- 1 teaspoon Vanilla
- 3 1/2 tablespoons Water
- Sprinkles optional

Directions

Air Fryer Donuts

1. To make a hole, open the biscuits and then use a small donut cutter.
2. Place the biscuit donuts at 350 degrees F on the lower rack in the air fryer, then cook for 3-4 minutes.
3. Flip the donuts, then fry for another 1 minute in the air.
4. Dip the donuts into the chocolate glaze and top as desired until it is cool enough to treat.

Chocolate Glaze

1. Combine the chocolate glaze components in a bowl and blend until mixed.
2. You can add 1 teaspoon of water at a time if it is too thick before it reaches the perfect consistency.

68. Strawberry Novella hand pies

Total time: 30 min

Prep time: 20 min

Cook time: 10 min

Yield: 8 servings

Ingredients

- 1 Pillsbury refrigerated pie crust
- 3 to 4 strawberries
- Novella
- sugar
- coconut oil cooking spray
- 3-inch heart cookie cutter

Directions

1. Unroll the crust of the pie. Using the knife as near as possible to cut out the hearts. Gather the scraps in a ball, thinly roll the ball out to get a few more heart shapes. For 8 hand pies, I was able to get 16 hearts out of one round pie crust.

2. Line a baking tray and set it aside with parchment paper.

3. Chop the strawberries finely and set them aside. Spread a dollop (about 1 teaspoon) of Novella on a single heart. Attach a few of the strawberry bits. Using a pinch of sugar to sprinkle.

4. Place another heart on top and use a fork to crimp the edges tightly. To gently poke holes in the top of the pie, use the fork. Turn to the baking tray.

5. On the plate, spray coconut oil on all of the pies. Shift the pies around the tray instead of tossing the pies to pick up additional coconut oil.

6. To cook in an air fryer, preheat the air fryer at 400 degrees F for 3 minutes. In the basket, put the pie hearts, making sure they don't hit each other. I managed to accommodate four of them at a time. Bake for 5 to 7 minutes or until browned properly. No need for hearts to flip.

7. Preheat to 400 degrees F for baking in an oven. Bake until well-browned, around 10 to 12 minutes on the baking tray.

69. Ube Glazed Air Fryer Donuts Recipe

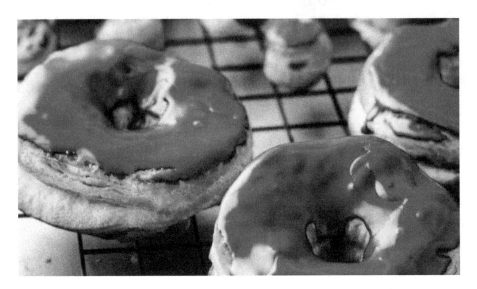

Total time: 11 min

Prep time: 5 min

Cook time: 6 min

Yield: 8 servings

Ingredients

- 1 cup powdered sugar
- 2 tablespoon milk
- 1/2 teaspoon use extract
- 1/4 teaspoon vanilla extract
- 1 can (16.3 ounces) Grands

Directions

1. Pre-heat a 350F air fryer.

2. Combine the powdered sugar, milk, use, and vanilla extract in a small cup. Whisk, until smooth, to mix.

3. Biscuits can be opened and placed on a cutting board. Cut out the middle hole of the donuts using a 1 inch round cookie cutter. To air dry, you can also hold the donut holes.

4. Spray the air fryer's basket with a non-stick cooking spray. Place donuts with room between each donut in the basket. When cooking, it's best not to stack these. These will need to be cooked in two batches. Three minutes of air-frying.

5. When you have up to three minutes, open the drawer and turn the donuts over. Close the drawer and fry for an additional 2 to 3 minutes.

6. Remove donuts and allow to cool slightly once air frying is complete. Then dip the donut into the glaze and allow it to cool completely over a cookie sheet on a wire cooling rack to catch excess drips. Enjoy

70. Apple Hand Pies

Total time: 25 min

Prep time: 10 min

Cook time: 15 min

Yield: 8 servings

Ingredients

- Pre Made Pie Crusts
- 5 oz. Can Apple Pie Filling
- 1 Egg

Directions

1. Roll out the crust of the pie and cut out circles using a cookie cutter.

2. Take half a spoonful of apple pie filling and put it in half of your circles in the middle of it.

3. Slightly roll out the remaining circles with a rolling pin, so they are a tab but larger than the apple circles.

4. Place the larger circle on the top and mend it together using a fork.

5. Wash every apple pie with an egg.

6. Place the air fryer at 350 degrees for 12-15 minutes.

7. Enjoy & serve

71. Air Fryer Beignets

Total time: 35 min

Prep time: 6 min

Cook time: 14 min

Yield: 9 servings

Ingredients

- 1 cup Self-Rising Flour
- 1 Cup Plain Greek Yogurt
- 2 TBSP Sugar
- 1 TSP Vanilla
- 2 TBSP Melted unsalted butter
- 1/2 Cup Powdered Sugar

Directions

1. In a cup, combine the yogurt, sugar & vanilla.

2. Put in the flour & stir until a dough begins to form.

3. On a floured surface, bring the dough on.

4. Fold the dough in half a couple of times.

5. Shape a rectangle 1 inch thick. Cut it into 9 bits. Dust each piece lightly with flour.

6. For 15 minutes, let them rest.

7. Preheat to 350 degrees with your air fryer.

8. Spray canola spray on your Air Fryer Tray/Basket.

9. Brush the melted butter on top of your dough.

10. On your tray or basket, put butter side down. Brush the dough tops with butter.

11. Air fry for approx. 6-7 minutes before brown begins on the edges.

12. Flip over and cook an extra 6-7 minutes.

13. Dust of sugar powder

72. Mini S'mores Pie

Total time: 8 min

Prep time: 2 min

Cook time: 6 min

Yield: 6 servings

Ingredients

- 6 Mini Graham Ready Crust

- 12 Snack Sized Hershey's Bars (broken in half)

- 1 Cup Mini Marshmallows

Directions

1. Pre-heat up to 320 degrees for your Air Fryer

2. Into each mini crust, put 4 broken pieces of Hershey strip.

3. You want enough of a top with mini marshmallows to fully cover your Hershey bars.

4. Air fry your marshmallows at 320 degrees for 5-7 minutes, depending on how toasty you like.

5. Serve & Enjoy immediately

73. Apple Pie Bombs

Total time: 21 min

Prep time: 5 min

Cook time: 16 min

Yield: 16 servings

Ingredients

- 1 cup apple pie filling
- 1 can Grands canned biscuits
- 1/2 cup butter
- 3/4 cup sugar
- 3 teaspoons ground cinnamon

Directions

1. Using a knife and a fork to cut the pie into small pieces.

2. Pull each of the biscuits into 2 layers and put them on a clean surface. Roll with a rolling pin to about a 4-inch circle or flatten with your fingertips.

3. Preheat the air fryer for 5 minutes to 350 °.

4. Fill each dough with a spoon and pull the sides together and pinch them to seal. Roll yourself into balls.

5. Place apple pie bombs about 2 inches apart in the air fryer basket, cooking in batches depending on how many of them you can fit into your basket.

6. Cook until golden brown or for 8 minutes.

7. Melt the butter as the first batch bakes.

8. Mix the sugar and cinnamon in a medium-sized dish.

9. Dip baked apple pie bombs on all sides in melted butter, letting the excess runoff.

10. Roll in the mixture of cinnamon sugar and put it on a wire rack.

11. With the remaining ingredients, repeat.

12. Serve at room temperature or instantly,

74. Baked Apples

Total time: 25 min

Prep time: 5 min

Cook time: 20 min

Yield: 4 servings

Ingredients

- 2 granny smith apples, halved and cored
- ¼ cup old fashioned oats (not the instant kind)
- 1 tbsp. butter, melted
- 2 tbsp. brown sugar
- ½ tsp. cinnamon
- Whipped cream for topping (optional

Directions

1. In the Air Fryer basket, lay cored apple halves in a single layer,

2. Air fry the plain apple halves for 10 minutes at 350 degrees.

3. Meanwhile, to form the topping, combine the oats, melted butter, brown sugar, and cinnamon.

4. Add topping to apple halves and continue air frying at 350 degrees for 5-10 more minutes until apples are tender and topping is crispy. Apples should be soft when you poke them in the center with a fork.

5. Serve warm and add whipped cream or ice cream optionally on the top.

75. Seafood Appetizer

Total time: 15 min

Prep time: 5min

Cook time: 10min

Yield: 2 serving

Ingredients:

- ½ cup of yellow onion, chopped
- 1 cup of green bell pepper, chopped
- 1 cup of celery, chopped
- 1 cup of baby shrimp, peeled and deveined
- 1 cup of crabmeat, flaked
- 1 cup of homemade mayonnaise
- 1 teaspoon of Worcestershire sauce
- Salt and black pepper to the taste
- 2 tablespoons of bread crumbs
- 1 tablespoon of butter
- 1 teaspoon of sweet paprika

Directions:

1. In a bowl, mix shrimp with crab meat, bell pepper, onion, mayo, celery, salt, pepper, and stir.

2. Add Worcestershire sauce, stir again, and pour everything into a baking dish that fits your Air Fryer.

3. Sprinkle bread crumbs and add butter, introduce in your Aurorae cook at 320° F for 25 minutes, shaking halfway.

4. Divide into a bowl and serve with paprika sprinkled on top as an appetizer.

Enjoy!

Nutrition: Calories: 200, Fat: 1g, Fiber: 2g, Carbs: 5g, Protein: 1g.

76. Salmon Meatballs

Total time: 15 min

Prep time: 5min

Cook time: 10min

Yield: 2 serving

Ingredients:

- 3 tablespoons of cilantro, minced
- 1-pound of salmon, skinless and chopped
- 1 small yellow onion, chopped
- 1 egg white
- Salt and black pepper to the taste
- 2 garlic cloves, minced
- ½ teaspoon of paprika
- ¼ cup of panko
- ½ teaspoon of oregano, ground
- Cooking spray

Directions:

1. Mix the salmon with the cabbage, cilantro, white egg, garlic cloves, salt, pepper, paprika, and oregano in your food processor and mix well.

2. Add panko, combine again and use your hands to form meatballs from this combination.

3. Place them in the basket of your Air Fryer, spray them with a cooking spray, and cook for 12 minutes at 320° F, shaking the fryer halfway.

4. Place meatballs on a platter and act as an appetizer.

77. Easy Chicken Wings

Total time: 15 min

Prep time: 5min

Cook time: 10min

Yield: 2 serving

Ingredients:

- 16 pieces ok chicken wings
- Salt and black pepper to the taste
- ¼ cup of butter
- ¾ cup of potato starch
- ¼ cup of honey
- 4 tablespoons of garlic, minced

Directions:

1. Mix the chicken wings with salt, pepper, and potato starch in a cup, mix well, move them to the basket of your Air Fryer, cook them for 25 minutes at 380° F, and 5 minutes more at 400° F.

2. In the meantime, prepare a buttered pan over medium-high heat, melt, add garlic, stir, simmer for 5 minutes, and then mix with salt, pepper, and honey.

3. Whisk well, cook for 20 minutes at medium pressure and take off-gas.

4. Arrange the chicken wings all over a pan, drizzle the honey sauce, and serve as an appetizer.

78. Chicken Breast Rolls

Total time: 15 min

Prep time: 5min

Cook time: 10min

Yield: 2 serving

Ingredients:

- 2 cups of baby spinach
- 4 chicken breasts, boneless and skinless
- 1 cup of sun-dried tomatoes, chopped
- Salt and black pepper to the taste
- 1 and ½ tablespoons of Italian seasoning
- 4 mozzarella slices
- A drizzle of olive oil

Directions:

1. Using a meat tenderizer to flatten the chicken breasts, split the tomatoes, mozzarella, spinach, season with salt, pepper, and Italian seasoning, roll, and close.

2. Place them in the basket of your Air Fryer, drizzle some oil over them, and cook for 17 minutes at 375° F, flipping once.

3. Arrange rolls of chicken on a pan, which serve as an appetizer.

79. Crispy Chicken Breast Sticks

Total time: 15 min

Prep time: 5min

Cook time: 10min

Yield: 2 serving

Ingredients:

- ¾ cup of white flour
- 1-pound chicken breast, skinless, boneless, and cut into medium sticks
- 1 teaspoon of sweet paprika
- 1 cup of panko bread crumbs
- 1 egg, whisked
- Salt and black pepper to the taste
- ½ tablespoon of olive oil
- Zest from 1 lemon, grated

Directions:

1. Mix the paprika in a bowl with the zest of flour, salt, pepper, lemon, and stir.

2. Placed the whisked egg in another bowl and the breadcrumbs panko in a seventh.

3. Dredge chicken parts in flour, egg, and panko, put them in the basket of your lined Air Fryer, drizzle the oil over them, cook for 8 minutes at 400° F, turn over and cook for another 8 minutes.

4. Put them up on a tray, and serve as a snack.

80. Beef Rolls

Total time: 15 min

Prep time: 5min

Cook time: 10min

Yield: 2 serving

Ingredients:

- 2 pounds of beef steak, opened and flattened with a meat tenderizer
- Salt and black pepper to the taste
- 1 cup of baby spinach
- 3 ounces of red bell pepper, roasted and chopped
- 6 slices of provolone cheese
- 3 tablespoons of pesto

Directions:

1. Arrange flattened beef steak on a cutting board, sprinkle pesto around, add cheese in a skillet, and add bell peppers, basil, salt, and pepper to taste.

2. Roll your beef, protect it with toothpicks, season again with salt and pepper, place the roll in your Air Fryer basket, and cook at 400 ° F for 14 minutes, slicing the roll in half.

3. Set aside to cool off, divide into smaller 2-inch rolls, arrange on a dish, and serve as an appetizer.

81. Empanadas

Total time: 15 min

Prep time: 5min

Cook time: 10min

Yield: 8 serving

Ingredients:

- One package of empanada shells
- 1 tablespoon of olive oil
- 1-pound beef meat, ground

- 1 yellow onion, chopped
- Salt and black pepper to the taste
- 2 garlic cloves, minced
- ½ teaspoon of cumin, ground
- ¼ cup of tomato salsa
- 1 egg yolk whisked with 1 tablespoon water
- 1 green bell pepper, chopped

Directions:

1. Heat a skillet over medium-high heat with the grease, add the beef, and brown on both sides.

2. Stir and simmer for 15 minutes; add onion, garlic, salt, vinegar, bell pepper, and tomato salsa.

3. Break the fried meat into shells of empanada, clean them with egg wash, and close.

4. Place these in the steamer basket of your Air Fryer and cook for 10 minutes at 350° F.

5. Arrange on a tray, and serve as an appetizer.

82. Greek Lamb Meatballs

Total time: 25 min

Prep time: 15min

Cook time: 10min

Yield: 8 serving

Ingredients:

- 4 ounces of lamb meat, minced
- Salt and black pepper to the taste
- 1 slice of bread, toasted and crumbled
- 2 tablespoons of feta cheese, crumbled
- ½ tablespoon of lemon peel, grated

- 1 tablespoon of oregano, chopped

Directions:

1. Combine meat in a bowl with crumbs of pasta, salt, pepper, feta, oregano, and lemon peel, stir well, shape 10 meatballs, and put them in your Air Fryer.

2. Cook for 8 minutes at 400° F, put them on a plate, and serve as an appetizer.

83. Beef Party Rolls

Total time: 25 min

Prep time: 15min

Cook time: 10min

Yield: 8 serving

Ingredients:

- 14 ounces of beef stock
- 7 ounces of white wine
- 4 beef cutlets
- Salt and black pepper to the taste
- 8 sage leaves
- 4 ham slices
- 1 tablespoon of butter, melted

Directions:

1. Heat a pan over medium heat with the stock, add wine, cook until it reduces, take off the heat, and separate into small bowls

2. Season the cutlets with salt and pepper, coat them with sage, and roll in slices of ham each.

3. Rub the rolls with butter, put them in the basket of your Air Fryer, and cook for 15 minutes at 400° F.

4. Arrange rolls on a pan, then serve them on the hand with the gravy.

84. Pork Rolls

Total time: 35 min

Prep time: 15min

Cook time: 20min

Yield: 8 serving

Ingredients:

- 15 ounce of pork fillet
- ½ teaspoon of chili powder
- 1 teaspoon of cinnamon powder
- 1 garlic clove, minced
- Salt and black pepper to the taste
- 2 tablespoons of olive oil
- 1 and ½ teaspoon of cumin, ground
- 1 red onion, chopped
- 3 tablespoons of parsley, chopped

Directions:

1. Mix the garlic, salt, pepper, chili powder, oil, onion, Petersen, and cumin with the cinnamon in a cup, and whisk well.

2. Place the pork fillet on a cutting board and use a meat tenderizer to flatten it. And flatten yourself with a beef tenderizer.

3. On the bacon, print the onion blend, roll tight, break into medium rolls, place it in your preheated Air Fryer at 360 ° F, and cook for 35 minutes.

4. Place them on a tray and look like an appetizer.

85. Masala French Fries

Total time: 27 min

Prep time: 10 min

Cook time: 17 min

Yield: 4 serving

Ingredients:

- 2 medium-sized potatoes peeled and cut into thick pieces lengthwise
- Ingredients for the marinade:
- 1 tbsp. of olive oil
- 1 tsp. of mixed herbs
- ½ tsp. of red chili flakes
- A pinch of salt to taste
- 1 tbsp. of lemon juice

Directions:

1. Break your fingertips into the onion, cook, and blanch the potatoes. Combine and add the potato fingers to the marinade ingredients, which ensures they are well fried.
2. Preheat the Air Fryer for about 5 minutes at 300 Fahrenheit. Take the bowl out of the fryer and put the potato fingers in it. Get the box closed. Even then, keep the fryer at 200 Fahrenheit for 20 to 25 minutes.
3. During the process, toss the fries two or three times so they'll be properly fried.

86. Dal Mint Kebab

Total time: 35 min

Prep time: 10 min

Cook time: 20 min

Yield: 2 serving

Ingredients:

- 1 cup of chickpeas
- Half inch ginger grated or one and a half tsp. of ginger-garlic paste
- 1-2 green chilies chopped finely
- ¼ tsp. of red chili powder
- A pinch of salt to the taste
- ½ tsp. of roasted cumin powder
- 2 tsp. of coriander powder
- 1 ½ tbsp. of chopped coriander
- ½ tsp. of dried mango powder
- 1 cup of dry breadcrumbs
- ¼ tsp. of black pepper
- 1-2 tbsp. of all-purpose flour for coating purposes
- 1-2 tbsp. of mint (finely chopped)
- 1 onion that has been finely chopped
- ½ cup of milk

Directions:

1. Take a yacht for free. Within the bowl, cook the chickpeas until they become smooth in texture. Make sure that they're not getting soggy. Now, in a different bowl, take your chickpea.

2. Apply the rubbed ginger and orange-sliced chilies. Grind the mixture until it turns into a paste that is smooth. Continue to add water as and when necessary. Now add the onions, mint, breadcrumbs, and all the various masalas that are required.

3. Mix until it is smooth for the pastry. Now, make small balls (about the size of a lemon) from this mix and mold them into a smooth, circular kebab shape. This is when it comes to milk. Spill a very small amount of milk onto each kebab to soak it. Fold the kebab into the dried bread crumbs now.

4. About 300 Fahrenheit, 5 minutes to preheat the Air Fryer. Let your bowl out. Arrange kebabs such that no two kebabs strike one another in the basket, leaving gaps in them. Hold the fryer, at 340 Fahrenheit, for almost half an hour.

5. Switch the kebabs over halfway through the process of cooking so they can be thoroughly fried. For this sauce, the chosen sides are mint chutney, tomato ketchup, or yogurt chutney.

87. Cottage Cheese Croquette

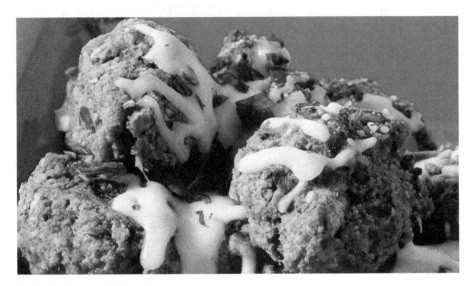

Total time: 25 min

Prep time: 10 min

Cook time: 15 min

Yield: 2 serving

Ingredients:

- 2 cups cottage cheese cut into slightly thick and long pieces (similar to French fries)
- 1 big capsicum (Cut this capsicum into big cubes)
- 1 onion (Cut it into quarters. Now separate the layers carefully.)
- 5 tbsp. of gram flour
- A pinch of salt to the taste

For chutney:

- 2 cups of fresh green coriander
- ½ cup of mint leaves

- 4 tsp. of fennel
- 1 small onion
- 2 tbsp. of ginger-garlic paste
- 6-7 garlic flakes (optional)
- 3 tbsp. of lemon juice
- Salt

Directions:

1. Take a tub that is dry and clean. Put in the coriander, basil, fennel, ginger, onion/garlic, salt, and lemon juice. Combine and complete.

2. Load the mixture into a grinder and then blend until it creates a smooth paste. So, move on to cottage cheese slices. Split almost to the edge of these pieces, then set them aside. Now, stuff all the bits with the paste from the previous process that was there. Set the boxed cottage cheese aside now.

3. Take the chutney and add to it some salt and some grams of flour. Mix all of them. Rub this mix all over the cottage cheese's stuffed bits. Set aside the cottage cheese now. Now add the remaining chutney with the capsicum and onions. Spread the chutney softly on top of the bits of capsicum and onion. Now, take satay sticks and place the cottage cheese bits and vegetables on separate sticks.

4. For about 5 minutes, preheat the Air Fryer at 290 Fahrenheit. Arrange the Satay holds correctly. Get the box closed. Hold the sticks with the cottage cheese at 180 ° for around half an hour, while the sticks with the vegetables should only be kept for 7 minutes at the same temperature.

5. Turn the sticks in between so that there is no burning on the one hand, and a daily cook is also provided.

88. Barbeque Corn Sandwich

Total time: 40 min

Prep time: 15 min

Cook time: 25 min

Yield: 2 serving

Ingredients:

- 2 slices of white bread
- 1 tbsp. of softened butter
- 1 cup of sweet corn kernels
- 1 small capsicum

For Barbeque Sauce:

- ¼ tbsp. of Worcestershire sauce
- ½ tsp. of olive oil
- ½ flake garlic crushed
- ¼ cup of chopped onion
- ¼ tbsp. of red chili sauce
- ½ cup of water

Directions:

1. Take the slices of bread, and the rims are sliced. On the strips, still cut horizontally. Heat up the spices for the sauce and wait until the sauce thickens. Now add the corn to the sauce and stir before receiving the flavors.

2. Whisk and clean off the skin with the capsicum. Sliced into strips is the capsicum. For the

trimmings, add the sauce. For 5 minutes, preheat the Air Fryer to Fahrenheit 300.

3. Open the basket of the fryer and drop the fried sandwiches in it, making sure that no two sandwiches touch each other. Hold the fryer at 250° for about 15 minutes.

4. Move the sandwiches between the two fires slice cooking processes. Serve the sandwiches with strawberry ketchup or mint chutney.

89. Bread Pudding

Total time: 25 min

Prep time: 5 min

Cook time: 20 min

Yield: 4 servings

Ingredients

- 2 cups bread cubed
- 1 egg
- 2/3 cup heavy cream
- 1/2 tsp. vanilla extract
- 1/4 cup sugar
- 1/4 cup chocolate chips optional

Directions

1. Spray with cooking spray on the inside of a baking dish that fits inside the air fryer.

2. In a baking dish, place cubes of bread. Sprinkle them over the bread if chocolate chips are used.

3. Mix the egg, whipped cream, vanilla and sugar in another dish.

4. Over the bread cubes, pour the egg mixture and let it stand for 5 minutes.

5. Within the air-fryer basket, place the baking dish. Cook for 15 minutes in the air fryer at 350F, or until the bread pudding is cooked through.

90. Beef Patties

Total time: 35 min

Prep time: 15min

Cook time: 20min

Yield: 8 serving

Ingredients:

- 14 ounces of beef, minced
- 2 tablespoons of ham, cut into strips
- 1 leek, chopped
- 3 tablespoons of bread crumbs
- Salt and black pepper to the taste
- ½ teaspoon of nutmeg, ground

Directions:

1. In a cup, blend beef and leek, salt, pepper, ham, breadcrumbs, and nutmeg, whisk well and turn this mixture into little patties.

2. Place them in your Air Fryer basket, cook at 400 ° F for 8 minutes, arrange them on a plate and serve them as an appetizer.

91. Roasted Bell Pepper Rolls

Total time: 20 min

Prep time: 10min

Cook time: 10min

Yield: 6 serving

Ingredients:

- 1 yellow bell pepper, halved
- 1 orange bell pepper, halved
- Salt and black pepper to the taste
- 4 ounces of feta cheese, crumbled
- 1 green onion, chopped
- 2 tablespoons of oregano, chopped

Directions:

1. In a cup, mix the cheese with the onion, oregano, salt, and pepper and whisk well.
2. Place the bell pepper halves in your Air Fryer basket, cook at 400 °F for 10 minutes, switch to a cutting board, cool down, and peel.
3. Break the cheese mixture into each half of the bell pepper, slice, secure with toothpicks, put on a tray, and serve as an appetizer.

92. Stuffed Peppers

Total time: 18 min

Prep time: 9min

Cook time: 9min

Yield: 6 serving

Ingredients:

- 8 small bell peppers, tops cut off and seeds removed
- 1 tablespoon of olive oil
- Salt and black pepper to the taste
- 3.5 ounces of goat cheese, cut into 8 pieces

Directions:

1. In a cup, add salt and pepper to the cheese and oil, and mix to cover.

2. Fill each pepper with goat cheese, put them in the basket of your Air Fryer, cook for 8 minutes at 400° F, arrange them on a platter and serve as an appetizer.

93. Herbed Tomatoes Appetizer

Total time: 18 min

Prep time: 9min

Cook time: 9min

Yield: 6 serving

Ingredients:

- 2 tomatoes, halved
- Cooking spray
- Salt and black pepper to the taste
- 1 teaspoon of parsley, dried
- 1 teaspoon of basil, dried
- 1 teaspoon of oregano, dried
- 1 teaspoon of rosemary, dried

Directions:

1. Sprinkle with cooking oil over the tomato halves and season with salt, pepper, parsley, basil, oregano, and rosemary.
2. Place these in your Air Fryer basket and cook at 320° F for 20 minutes.
3. Put them up to serve as an appetizer on a plate.

94. Olives Balls

Total time: 18 min

Prep time: 9min

Cook time: 9min

Yield: 6 serving

Ingredients:

- 8 black olives, pitted and minced
- Salt and black pepper to the taste
- 2 tablespoons of sun-dried tomato pesto
- 14 pepperoni slices, chopped
- 4 ounces of cream cheese
- 1 tablespoon of basil, chopped

Directions:

1. Mix the cream cheese with salt, pepper, basil, pepperoni, pesto, and black olives in a cup, stir well, and make small balls out of the mixture.

2. Place them in the basket of your Air Fryer, cook for 4 minutes at 350° F, arrange them on a plate and serve as a snack.

113. Jalapeno Balls

Total time: 18 min

Prep time: 9min

Cook time: 9min

Yield: 6 serving

Ingredients:

- 3 bacon slices, cooked and crumbled
- 3 ounces of cream cheese
- ¼ teaspoon of onion powder
- Salt and black pepper to the taste
- 1 jalapeno pepper, chopped

- ½ teaspoon of parsley, dried
- ¼ teaspoon of garlic powder

Directions:

1. In a cup, combine the cream cheese, jalapeno paste, onion and garlic powder, parsley, bacon, salt, and pepper and blend well.

2. Shape tiny balls out of this mix, put them in your Air Fryer basket, cook at 350 ° F for 4 minutes, place them on a dish and serve as an appetizer.

95. Wrapped Shrimp

Total time: 18 min

Prep time: 9min

Cook time: 9min

Yield: 16 serving

Ingredients:

- 2 tablespoons of olive oil
- 10 ounces of already cooked shrimp, peeled and deveined
- 1 tablespoon of mint, chopped
- 1/3 cup of blackberries, ground
- 11 prosciuttos sliced
- 1/3 cup of red wine

Directions:

1. Wrap each shrimp into a slice of prosciutto, drizzle the oil over them, rub well, put 390° F in your preheated Air Fryer and fry them for 8 minutes.

2. In the meantime, fire up a skillet over medium heat with ground blackberries, add mint and juice, mix, simmer for 3 minutes and take off the heat.

3. Place shrimp on a platter, sauce blackberries over them, and serve as an appetizer.

96. Broccoli Patties

Total time: 18 min

Prep time: 9min

Cook time: 9min

Yield: 12 serving

Ingredients:

- 4 cups of broccoli florets
- 1 and ½ cup of almond flour
- 1 teaspoon of paprika
- Salt and black pepper to the taste
- 2 eggs
- ¼ cup of olive oil
- 2 cups of cheddar cheese, grated
- 1 teaspoon of garlic powder
- ½ teaspoon of apple cider vinegar
- ½ teaspoon of baking soda

Directions:

1. In your food processor, place broccoli florets, add salt and pepper, blend well, and move to a dish.

2. Add the almond flour, cinnamon, pepper, paprika, garlic powder, baking soda, butter, milk, eggs, and vinegar, blend well, and form 12 patties from this mixture.

3. Place them in the basket of your preheated Air Fryer and cook for 10 minutes at 350° F.

4. Place patties on a pan, and act as an appetizer.

118. Different Stuffed Peppers

Total time: 18 min

Prep time: 9min

Cook time: 9min

Yield: 12 serving

Ingredients:

- 1-pound mini bell peppers halved
- Salt and black pepper to the taste
- 1 teaspoon of garlic powder
- 1 teaspoon of sweet paprika
- ½ teaspoon of oregano, dried
- ¼ teaspoon of red pepper flakes
- 1-pound beef meat, ground
- 1 and ½ cups of cheddar cheese, shredded
- 1 tablespoon of chili powder
- 1 teaspoon of cumin, ground
- Sour cream for serving

Directions:

1. Mix the chili powder with paprika, salt, pepper, cumin, oregano, pepper flakes, and garlic powder in a cup and stir.

2. Heat a medium pressure casserole, add beef, stir and brown for 10 minutes.

3. Add the chili powder mixture, stir, remove from the heat and add half the pepper to the mixture.

4. Sprinkle the cheese all over, drop the peppers in your Air Fryer basket and roast them at 350 ° F for 6 minutes.

5. On a tray, arrange the peppers, then eat them vertically with sour cream.

97. Cheesy Zucchini Snack

Total time: 18 min

Prep time: 9min

Cook time: 9min

Yield: 12 serving

Ingredients:

- 1 cup of mozzarella, shredded
- ¼ cup of tomato sauce
- 1 zucchini, sliced
- Salt and black pepper to the taste
- A pinch of cumin
- Cooking spray

Directions:

1. Arrange the zucchini slices in the basket of your Air Fryer, spray them with cooking oil, scatter the tomato sauce all over, season them with salt, pepper, cumin, sprinkle the mozzarella at the end, and roast them for 8 minutes at 320° F.

2. Put them up on a tray and serve as a snack.

98. Spinach Balls

Total time: 30 min

Prep time: 15min

Cook time: 15

Yield: 30 serving

Ingredients:

- 4 tablespoons of butter, melted
- 2 eggs
- 1 cup of flour
- 16 ounces of spinach
- 1/3 cup of feta cheese, crumbled
- ¼ teaspoon of nutmeg, ground
- 1/3 cup of parmesan, grated
- Salt and black pepper to the taste
- 1 tablespoon of onion powder
- 3 tablespoons of whipping cream
- 1 teaspoon of garlic powder

Directions:

1. In your mixer, add the spinach with the butter, sugar, spaghetti, feta cheese, parmesan cheese, nutmeg, whipped cream, salt, pepper, onion and garlic powder, mix really well, and freeze for 10 minutes.
2. Shape 30 balls of spinach, drop them in your Air Fryer basket and cook at 300 °F for 7 minutes.
3. Serve to an audience like an appetizer.

99. Mushrooms Appetizer

Total time: 30 min

Prep time: 15min

Cook time: 15

Yield: 30 serving

Ingredients:

- ¼ cup of mayonnaise
- 1 teaspoon of garlic powder

- 1 small yellow onion, chopped
- 24 ounces of white mushroom caps
- Salt and black pepper to the taste
- 1 teaspoon of curry powder
- 4 ounces of cream cheese, soft
- ¼ cup of sour cream
- ½ cup of Mexican cheese, shredded
- 1 cup of shrimp, cooked, peeled, deveined, and chopped

Directions:

1. In a bowl of garlic powder, onion, curry powder, cream cheese, sour cream, Mexican cheese, seafood, salt, and pepper, combine the mayo and shake well.
2. Place the mushrooms with this mixture in your Air Fryer basket and cook at 300 ° F for 10 minutes.
3. Arrange and serve as an appetizer on a tray.

100. Cheesy Party Wings

Total time: 22 min

Prep time: 11min

Cook time: 11

Yield: 6 serving

Ingredients:

- 6-pound chicken wings halved
- Salt and black pepper to the taste
- ½ teaspoon of Italian seasoning
- 2 tablespoons of butter
- ½ cup parmesan of cheese, grated

- A pinch of red pepper flakes, crushed
- 1 teaspoon of garlic powder
- 1 egg

Directions:

1. Arrange the chicken wings in your Air Fryer tray and bake at 390° F for 9 minutes.

2. Meanwhile, in your mixer, add the butter with cheese, milk, salt, pepper, pepper flakes, garlic powder, and Italian seasoning and mix well.

3. Take out chicken wings, spill over the cheese sauce, mix well to coat, and cook at 390 ° F. Serve them like an appetizer in your Air Fryer's basket for 3 minutes.

4. Cut the onions and peppers into thin slices while the chicken is frying. In a wok, apply the olive oil and cook for a minute over medium-high heat. Toss all the vegetables together and sauté for five minutes.

5. Mix the fish sauce, oyster sauce, hot chili sauce, soy sauce, and mix well for 1 minute. Apply the basil and chicken leaves and whisk until the leaves are wilted.

6. Serve over jasmine rice.

Conclusion

Unlike conventional deep-fryers, since they do not need to be soaked in oil, air fryers do not need oil. With the food being placed in first, they need only the right amount of oil between the food products. The deep-frying procedure in oil is a dangerous threat to health as it can cause heart attacks and other risks for individuals who eat a lot of this oily food. This possibility has been minimized by the air fryer.

CPSIA information can be obtained
at www.ICGtesting.com
Printed in the USA
BVHW062042010321
601387BV00007B/325